"Cures"

"CURES"

Medical Experts don't want to admit to

Compilation of Writings from:

Duke Bishop Captain Sir

Dr. William B. Mount, (U.S. Army, Retired)

and

Sir Dr. William P. Wilson

Edited by: Sir Pat JHS and Sir Keith Ljunghammar

Introduction by Sir Pat JHS

William B. Mount

Library of Congress Control Number:		2015902229
ISBN:	Hardcover	978-1-5035-3833-7
	Softcover	978-1-5035-3832-0
	eBook	978-1-5035-3831-3

AudioBook available also.

Print information available on the last page.

Rev. date: 09/08/2015

To order additional copies of this book, contact:
Xlibris
1-888-795-4274
www.Xlibris.com
Orders@Xlibris.com
686413

Dedicated to:

Thanking the I AM that I AM for giving Dr. Mount suggestions and guidance in his research in trying to find out how the body can heal itself.

Contents

Introduction to Healing

By Sir Pat Shupe

Cancer/Aids/Diabetes planned Population Control What The Public Knows of the Truth about Cancer

The Real Truth About Cancer, Aids, Diabetes and the complete Regenerative Capability of the Human Body by understanding some simple observations that have been kept from your understanding via for example cancer, aids and diabetes cannot exist in an a body that is alkaline and will simply just go away if the person simply changes their dietary habits and drinking habits and directs their body to becoming simply alkaline.

Read the following and realize How Really Big the Big Scam by Elitists Really is to Mass Murder You, Your Families, Your Communities, and Your Nation, Off while solely and only they and their globalist money laundering corporate network reaps in vast profiteering from your dying for them. Nothing like dying for the Globalist Elitist Satanist Luciferian Scheme of Destiny is there?

Some day the future of Medicine will be based on what will be considered to be "the physics of enzymes" or thereof the meaning of all life as we consider it scientifically as that of being the future until that day the Global Elitists will continue to utilize their complete control over the planet's entire system of medicine for only their sole profiteering agendas while utilizing their complete control over all education and media to manipulate and to dumb down the trusting sheeples supported with their systems of mass eliminations, mind control, and fluoridation and that the sheeples currently are mentally programmed to think is good for them when all that it does is destroy the brains of the sheeples and dumb them down so that they cannot see what is controlling and destroying their destiny.

The Elitists implemented diabetes via in part by forcing their sedentary salt "Morton Salt" that has less than 9 parts per million of in-organic minerals whereas Sea Salt has well over 120 parts per million heliotropic solar charged organic minerals and whereas it has been fully verified that sedentary mineral (Morton) salt does play a key part in shutting down the pancreas whereas sea salt actually heals the pancreas. When the pancreas shuts down it cannot any longer properly balance the serotonin, the enzymes in the blood and the ionic balance of the immune system let alone assist in keeping the body's immune system in an alkaline state where cancer, aids and diabetes cannot thus exist in a naturally alkaline bio system. Until the sheeples wake up to this very simple means of understanding as to how to heal themselves of all cancer, aids, and diabetes and as to why they have been misled by the Elitists who have created their fast food industries for heavy metal acid food waste bombardment of the human bio system that increases there: cancer, diabetes, aids medical industry monopoly mass profiteering scam for solely their own implemented mass human population control while they make the profits off of the dumbed down populations who cannot or will not figure this out.

A person who was scheduled to die within a month evidently tried out this solution and drank it every two hours and today is thriving and vitally alive with no known cancers in their body and this was more than ten years ago. They evidently also did the toxic removal methodology routine by also taking cayenne pepper - capsicum red pepper capsule thus converting their bio-system to becoming alkaline and non acidic as is described effectively by Dr. Len Horowitz.

Dr. Len Horowitz.

https://www.google.com/search?q=Dr.+Len+Horowitz&ie=utf-8&oe=utf-8&aq=t&rls=org.mozilla:en-US:official&client=firefox-a

Brown's Gas "Super Healing Water"

Posted by Will P. Wilson the producer of the All Day Live TV show and appears on Call4Investigation program that appear weekly on Seattle Community Media (***http://www.SeattleCommunityMedia.com*** **- & linked from *http://www.MediaCific.com*)**

All Day Live TV program is covering an interview with Dawn Darington concerning a DEA Cease and Desist Order that had been issued on Friday,

August 24, 2012 to the Medical Cannabis Clinic Choice Wellness (http://www.ChoiceWellnessWA.com) and this order was also issued to (Dawn Darington). (Shortly after this the popular vote made Cannabis legal in Washington State.)

Choice Wellness is a Medical Cannabis Access Point and a holistic Medical Facility that is located in the University of Washington District of Seattle. (Huge amount of research and personal testimony will conclusively indicate to most anyone that Cannabis has been proven over and over to have tremendous healing capabilities in its various forms of proper use.)

Reference and on-line links to this All Day Program: Dawn-Darington, Bruce-Perlowin, Hemp Inc., Cannabis-Industry, Medical-Cannabis, Seattle-Hempfest, King-of-Pot, Washington-State-Cannabis-Legislation, *http://www.Marijuana-Inc.tv. http://www.HempInc.tv, http://www.ChoiceWellnessWA.com*
(August 30, 2012) - http://seattlecommunitymedia.org/series/all-day-live/episode/all-day-live-willpwilson-mediacificcom-dawn-darington-choicewellnesswabr

AllDayLive Bruce Perlowin

https://www.google.com/search?q=alldaylive+Bruce+Perlowin&ie=utf-8&oe=utf-8&aq=t&rls=org.mozilla:en-US:official&client=firefox-a

How to Heal severed appendages

Add one ounce of DMSO - Dimethyl sulfoxide

-http://en.wikipedia.org/wiki/Dimethyl_sulfoxide

https://www.google.com/search?q=DMSO&ie=utf-8&oe=utf-8&aq=t&rls=org.mozilla:en-US:official&client=firefox-a

Dr. Stanley Jacobs DMSO

https://www.google.com/search?q=Dr.+Stanley+Jacobs+DMSO&ie=utf-8&oe=utf-8&aq=t&rls=org.mozilla:en-US:official&client=firefox-a

Add one ounce of MSM - Dr. Stanley Jacobs MSM

https://www.google.com/search?q=Dr.+Stanley+Jacobs+MSM&ie=utf-8&oe=utf-8&aq=t&rls=org.mozilla:en-US:official&client=firefox-a

Add two ounces of Colloidal Silver Water

https://www.google.com/search?q=Colloidal+Silver+Water&ie=utf-8&oe=utf-8&aq=t&rls=org.mozilla:en-US:official&client=firefox-a

Add two ounces of Colloidal Gold Water

https://www.google.com/search?q=Colloidal+Gold+Water&ie=utf-8&oe=utf-8&aq=t&rls=org.mozilla:en-US:official&client=firefox-a

Add two ounces of food grade 42% Hydrogen Peroxide

https://www.google.com/search?q=food+grade+42%25+Hydrogen+Peroxide&ie=utf-8&oe=utf-8&aq=t&rls=org.mozilla:en-US:official&client=firefox-a

Then I let this sit over night and until I was able to visit with this person the next day. I then arrived at this person's home and I proceeded to sit with them and to provide them with this soaking solution so that they might be able to heal their fingers more quickly than usual.

They then listened to me describe to them how they can place their surgically re-attached fingers in the solution but that it was not under my advice and that they must decide to go forward to do this.

But the person did decide to soak their re-attached fingers in this solution and I suggested that they do this procedure every two hours for at least fifteen minutes and preferably a half hour each time.

So I sat with this person for about two hours and they had decided to proceed with this soaking and within the first few minutes they mentioned that the bones of their fingers were aching and I realized that the regeneration of their fingers had begun.

So I left that Saturday around one. Then I was contacted by this person the next Thursday to come over to their home as soon as possible.

So I went over to their residence where the person hugged me and slapped my back with the hand that had the severed fingers only a few days before.

This person's fingers had completely regenerated within five days with no scar, with complete movement and the person mentioned that the surgical team thought that the re-attached fingers surgery team had pulled off a miracle.

Well, in a sense they had pulled off a miracle, but remember that our entire corporate medical system is completely controlled by what one can only consider to be an alleged corporate international fascist crime syndicate.

It will be soon discovered that this amazing catalyst water will be found to be able to remove nuclear contamination from the human body. And, as well as Medical Cannabis and Medical Mycology - (Mycology is the study of mushrooms) will also be discovered to not only be able to remove nuclear contamination from the human body but to also cure cancer, psoriasis, and possibly MRSA (Methicillin-resistant Staphylococcus aureus (MRSA) infection), and Morgellons Disease and possibly also help people during a biological-neurological warfare outbreak of some kind.

Mycology

https://www.google.com/search?q=Mycology&ie=utf-8&oe=utf-8&aq=t&rls=org.mozilla:en-US:official&client=firefox-a

Medical Mycology

https://www.google.com/search?q=medical+mycology&ie=utf-8&oe=utf-8&aq=t&rls=org.mozilla:en-US:official&client=firefox-a

Medical Cannabis

https://www.google.com/search?q=Medical+Cannabis&ie=utf-8&oe=utf-8&aq=t&rls=org.mozilla:en-US:official&client=firefox-a

MSRA

https://www.google.com/search?q=MSRA&ie=utf-8&oe=utf-8&aq=t&rls=org.mozilla:en-US:official&client=firefox-a

Morgellons disease
https://www.google.com/search?q=morgellons+disease&ie=utf-8&oe=utf-8&aq=t&rls=org.mozilla:en-US:official&client=firefox-a

http://www.apfn.net/Messageboard/09-28-06/discussion.cgi.50.html

Chapter One

Brown's Gas "Super Healing Water"

By Sir Dr. Will P. Wilson

Someday in the future, it will be also discovered that the very cells of our human bodies are literally producers of "Brown's Gas" and are held together by "Brown's Gas." That this gas that is only comprised of being *66.6 percent hydrogen, 33.3 percent oxygen,* created from only water that is produced by simple low voltage will also weld anything to anything, heal all known diseases, regenerate the human body to be enabled to live for literally hundreds of years, neutralize all nuclear waste material, power all piston engine technology, replace the oil energy industry for forever and that it will someday play a key part in literally helping mankind to discover new forms of elements, materials and to help mankind build non chemical utilizing means of travel beyond the stars using "Gyroscopic Aether Technology."

http://disc.yourwebapps.com/discussion.cgi?disc=149495;article=124858

The later discoveries about regenerative capabilities evidently revealed that this combined solution will cure all or most diseases as with the Dr. Willard's Catalyst Altered Water. When used as a solution catalyst it will increase not only the cellular oxidation factor by several hundred percent but also accelerate the absorption of co-mixed additives like MSM up to a thousand times and regenerate the human body to being longevity sustainable and approximate regenerative reversing of the aging process to twenty years younger or more. This solution could be a means of leading to the discovery of human immortality as said by one researcher.

Another person who was scheduled to die within a month evidently tried out this solution and drank it every two hours and today is thriving and vitally alive with no known cancers in their body and this was more than ten years ago. They evidently also did the toxic removal methodology routine by taking cayenne pepper - capsicum red pepper capsule thus converting their bio-system to becoming alkaline and non acidic as is described effectively by Dr. Len Horowitz.

Dr. Len Horowitz

https://www.google.com/search?q=Dr.+Len+Horowitz&ie=utf-8&oe=utf-8&aq=t&rls=org.mozilla:en-US:official&client=firefox-a

Some day the future of Medicine will be based on what will be considered to be "the physics of enzymes" or thereof the meaning of all life as we consider it scientifically as that of being the future development and understanding of: "Catalytic Ionic Physics" whereas until that day, the Global Elitists will continue to utilize their complete control over the planet's entire system of medicine for only their sole profiteering agendas while utilizing their complete control over all education and media to manipulate and to dumb down the trusting sheeples supported with their systems of mass eliminations, mind control, and fluoridation and that the sheeples currently are mentally programmed to think is good for them when all that it does is destroy the brains of the sheeples and dumb them down so that they cannot see what is controlling and destroying their destiny.

The Elitists implemented diabetes via in part by forcing their sedentary salt "Morton Salt" that has less than 9 parts per million of in-organic minerals whereas Sea Salt has well over 120 parts per million heliotropic solar charged organic minerals and whereas it has been fully verified that sedentary mineral (Morton) salt does play a key part in shutting down the pancreas whereas sea salt actually heals the pancreas. When the pancreas shuts down it cannot any longer properly balance the serotonin, the enzymes in the blood and the ionic balance of the immune system let alone assist in keeping the body's immune system in an alkaline state where cancer, aids and diabetes cannot thus exist in a naturally alkaline bio system. Until the sheeples wake up to this very simple means of understanding as to how to heal themselves of all cancer, aids, and diabetes and as to why they have been misled by the Elitists who have created their fast food industries for heavy metal acid food waste bombardment of the human bio system that increases there: cancer, diabetes, aids medical industry monopoly mass profiteering scam for solely their own implemented mass human population control while they make the profits off of the dumbed-down populations who cannot or will not figure this out.

Brown's Gas Heals

http://www.google.com/search?hl=en&lr=&q=Browns+Gas+Water+heals&btnG=Search

They saw Brown's Gas being used to heal people's bodies and taste Brown's Gas enhanced water.

http://www.eagle-research.com/newsletter/archive/2003/2003_02.html

Results 1 - 10 of about 15,900,000 for Browns Gas Water helps.

http://www.google.com/search?hl=en&sa=X&oi=spell&resnum=0

&ct=result&cd=1&q=Browns+Gas+Water+helps&spell=1

http://www.eagle-research.com/browngas/fabuses/possib.html

- *hydrated water for health*

When Brown's Gas is bubbled through clean water, the water absorbs oxygen and hydrogen. We think there is an additional energy (electrical in nature) added to the water as well. We find the drinking of the resulting enhanced, oxygenated and hydrated water to bring us to an alert state like drinking a cup of coffee, without the side effects.

Many people know that oxygenated water is healthful. There are many companies selling water that has had oxygen added to it.

What is generally unknown is that water is even more healthful when hydrogen is added to it. Drinking water is called hydrating the body. An astonishing fact is that chlorinated water, coffee, carbonated and sweetened fluids are generally dehydrating. Most of the diseases known to mankind (including aging) can be prevented or mitigated by hydrating the body.

Every test of Brown's Gas enhanced water shows it to be super hydrating, far superior to regular water (as much as 10 times).

Enhanced water is an essential key to keeping an active youthful body as the years go by.

We have reason to believe this water enhances every chemical process in the body, making a super immune system and mitigating the symptoms of aging, mostly caused by dehydration.

- detoxifying water - In North America chlorine is used to purify water, intending to kill microorganisms that cause disease. Chlorine is a deadly poison and attempts are made to put in just enough to kill the microorganisms and not the person drinking it. Most of the rest of the world purifies water using Ozone.

Thank you, Sir Dr. William P. Wilson for the contribution of this Chapter on Brown's Gas.

Chapter Two

How to Cure AGENT ORANGE Exposure

This is perhaps one of the hardest things to do - but it can be done.

First: Remember that when you are filing for Agent Orange Exposure you say: I do not know what I was exposed to exactly - but here is what happened to me and here is the documentation to prove it."

1) Never claim you were exposed to Agent Orange - just "Sprayed with something."
   Otherwise you will lose the case.

2) Always apply for disability through a Service Organization - never directly through the VA.

   I like our local DAV and American Legion office.

3) How to get rid of Agent Orange, Dioxin and other contaminants: See: The Cure for Cancer, Update 3, (Chapter 7, page 50)

Also use Immusist.com.

The Ion Cleanse, the Immusist and the green tea will clean you out pretty well in about 3 years.

Do not stop treating yourself for cancer either.

One last thing - the best topical ointment I have found for Jungle Rot is Oregano Oil. Hands Down.

We are also experimenting with Immusist.

If some Federal Agency pulls these products off the market we have 100 waiting in the wings to take their places - especially Immusist.

They are cheaper but perhaps a little less effective.

Chapter Three

The Cure for ALZHEIMER

This is one of the scariest diseases we could ever encounter. We literally loose our ability to remember even who we are.

We all have watched some loved one slip away from us day to day only to die in some rest home after they forget who we are.

It tears us apart to see Aunt Judy or you own mom to have to go through this.

Did you know that in 95% of the cases not only can we stop it's progression but reverse it?

1) Where does it come from?

There are 4 causes we can attribute this to:

a) In the early 1980's Mad Cow Disease was released just outside the British Weapons Lab. The cows got sick so they slaughtered them. As is normally done - the brains are turned into liquid and sprayed on cattle feed, sold around the world.

Within weeks this disease had literally been spread around the world by those in the British Bio-Weapons Lab.

Alzheimer rates skyrocketed.

The Mad Cow Disease vibrates when it gets near Aluminum - and this vibration tears off the protective coating that surrounds the nerve cells - and you get stupid.

Holes literally develop in your brain so you get Stubborn and pretend nothing is happening as your brain shrinks.

Over one third of all American's over 65 have this horrible disease.

b) Lyme Disease. 70% of all Alzheimer patients are positive for this disease - a gift from the US Bio Weapons Lab. This is another Nerve destroying virus.

c) Vaccinations. The heavy Metals are designed to destroy our nerves at around age 60 as the chemical make up in our body changes.

Sneaky of these vaccines companies, isn't it?

d) The eating of human Flesh. Read APFN SOILENT GREEN. When we eat Human Meat our Codon 127 changes to Codon 129 and we this assures us we will get Alzheimer's disease. Over 50% of all American's test positive for Codon 129.

Rapid Scanners at the Airports were purchased to support their parent company which - well - you figure out the rest. They make Soylent Green and we eat it.

e) There is a small percentage (5%) that just gets old.

2) So what is the cure?

First, as in all other articles - it can be reversed in 95% of the cases - but you will need to continue to follow the protocol for the rest of your life. The patient must be willing to listen - and that is the hard part.

Part of Alzheimer is they become Stubborn - angry, unwilling to change.

Please see: APFN THE CURE FOR CANCER, UPDATE 3 (Chapter 7, page 50) and begin following these protocols to detoxify the body and bring nutrition into your patient.

So here is what every clinician has told me around the country in private communications: A Solution of 25 MG Testosterone once per day reverses 95% of all Alzheimer disease in 90 days Period.

That is pretty darn impressive, right?

This can be obtained from one "Androgel packets" daily from Abbot Laboratories.

It works well on Women as well - but they grow a beard. We recommend you send women to a doctor that can prescribe Progesterone and the other hormones to help her. It is the Progesterone that reverses the Alzheimer disease - but Women have really complicated hormones - so go to a Hormone Doctor.

You see - these moderate doses of Hormones simply re-grow the nerves in the brain.

I do recommend looking at treating them for Lyme disease - and Mad Cow Disease. These diseases can be contained using the same methods outlined here in: APFN THE CURE FOR HIV (Chapter 13, page 73) - or in: APFN THE CURE FOR LYME DISEASE (Chapter 14, page 78).

It is not Rocket Science and it works.

This 95% reversal in 90 days, has repeated over and over again in clinic after clinic.

In my experience - the other 5% do not want to come back - and you must accept their decision no matter how hard it seems at the time. It is hard though, it brings allot of tears and soul searching - but you must accept them for who they are. I understand personally.

Someday someone will take these ideas and publish a book on it - I hope they make millions.

Freely I received - so freely I give - especially to our veterans.

Chapter Four

Cure for ARTHRITIS, UPDATE 1

As you recall we published the Cure for Arthritis.

We follow the same protocols as in: APFN THE CURE FOR CANCER, UPDATE 3 (Chapter 7, page 50) and Cure for Diabetes, (Chapter 9, page 61).

We
1) Detoxify
2) Kill the bad bugs and bring in the good bugs
3) Provide Proper Nutrition.

In most cases the progression of Arthritis is stopped with additional Iodine.

We have a friend named "Carol." Her Arthritis is so very bad her toes had to be surgically straightened and she cannot use the Ion Cleanse Machine to detoxify.

About 1 month ago we brought her some Immusist - see Immusist.com.

One month later - not only is she back to driving but she can begin to function as a normal human being. I have known her for about 8 years now and she has improved so much she is doing better than she was 8 years ago.

Carol is about 65 years old and 1 year ago was almost completely crippled and beginning to forget everything because of the drugs the Doctor's have prescribed her.

Now Carol is president of out local Solar Group and able to make her appointments every time. Shopping is a breeze now.

APFN readers - doesn't it give you great pleasure - excitement to be part of things like this?

Does it not send chills down your spine when you hear about a 65 year old woman who now is literally losing her Arthritis and pain?

Next Week we will do another scan on her Arteries leading to the brain to see if these procedures are actually clearing out her arteries of Plaque.

Pray that those who need to be cured of Arthritis read this article and act on it so as to alleviate their pain and not be crippled.

Chapter Five

Cause of AUTISM

We all know what the US is trying to do - these leaders are literally trying to destroy not only America but the rest of the world as well.

We are being assaulted on all fronts - Food, water, vaccinations, economy, socially, etc.

There are so many U.S. Army regulations and new laws allowing the opening of FEMA camps all across America and Canada.

This series of articles about "The Cure" are intended to help those who wish to not only survive but thrive in the near future.

See article: "Monkeys get Autism Like Reactions to MMR and other vaccines in University of Pittsburg Vaccine study." 29 April 2012.

Dr Laura Hewiston of the University of Pittsburg injected Macaque Monkeys with the Measles-Mumps-Rubella (MMR) vaccines and other vaccines containing high levels of Thimerosal (Mercury) - the same ones Mandated to give children - and a whole lot of monkeys became autistic.

Surprised?

Did anyone on Congress, or the FBI, or US Department of Justice or FDA or Any Federal Agency mandating Vaccinations listen? No.

To date there are no known Verifiable Government studies by the CDC, FDA, etc. on the effects of Multiple Vaccinations of Children. Period.

In fact, children who "appear autistic" went from 1/5,000 in 1990 to 1/6 today thanks to these same Government agencies, although many are simply classified with "Learning Disabilities."

You are injecting Biological and Chemical agents into your baby -you are killing it - Now you know!

What it boils down to is this: David Rothschild - who owns 54.5% of the IMF - which owns the US (See Senate Report 93-549) works for Lucifer and wants you dead.

((((Agents like Creep Perverted Governor Rick Snyder are following orders and destroying farmers and farmland purposely because he is also a Perverted Agent of Lucifer.)))))))

That is right - one in 6 children have learning difficulties and this can be traced right back to the day they received a Vaccination.

We have several children in the local Autism Group that were walking and talking and 2-3 days after receiving a Vaccination "MAGICALLY" became autistic.

Gee - how did that happened, I wonder?

Moms - stop making your babies Autistic.

If you want your child to live - do not use vaccinations.

If you want to cure a disease see: WILLIAM MOUNT THE CURE FOR HIV (Chapter 13, page 73).

If you want to cure Cancer see: APFN THE CURE FOR CANCER, UPDATE 3 (Chapter 7, page 50).

If you want to cure Heart Disease see: APFN THE CURE FOR HEART DISEASE (Chapter 12, page 67).

If you want to change things then get off the stick and start calling folks. Turn off the radio (Except Coast to Coast and El Rushbo, throw the TV away and get involved or be destroyed. It is that simple.

So there you have it - a Published, documented University study that clear and unopposed study, that shows US Vaccinations CAUSE Autism.

If you want to cure Autism see: WILLIAM MOUNT THE CAUSE OF AUTISM (and Chapter 5, page 30) or: APFN THE CURE FOR AUTISM (and Chapter 5, updates 1, 2, 3, 4, pages 35-47).

For You Intel Geeks:

1) There has been a lot of speculation about this "Super Moon" causing earthquakes. Earthquakes will occur when GOD says they will occur, and not one minute before then.
   As for the folks who are doing this research - your work is solid and we all appreciate what you do.

You want Big Earthquakes - then let a new series start NOW and last for a week, so says the I AM That I AM.

2) As for the U.S. Politicians who just told President Putin it does not matter because the world is about to end: It will end when GOD says it will.

GOD has already stated the Sun will get very bad very fast unless the leaders of this world do as he instructs.

This has not changed one iota.

As for Nostradamus's predictions: His strange way of speaking left many to predict the end of the world dozens of times in the last 450 years. He was a master of Gibberish. He twists words to mean almost anything.

If GOD says there will be an earthquake in 2 days - there will be one in 2 days. GOD is very specific and those of you who have read my APFN article know this.

3) A note to the USAF: You screwed up 2,000 Mother boards on Nuke. Good luck finding them and fixing them.

4) One last comment: As the quakes begin on Earth they will also begin on Mars - there is no place to run, no place to hide. Either follow GOD and do as HE asks - you know, the 10 commandments - or prepare your obituary, so says the I AM That I AM, who was and is and is to come.

Pray - Visualize - that Sam Baker stomps the Creepy Perverted Governor of Michigan ASAP. If Sam wins it will protect small farms everywhere.

Pray - Visualize - That you find your way through what is coming.

You Deserve the Truth

Honorable Grace
Dr William B. Mount
Knight of Malta
pt (En) USA
William Mount
Monkeys get Autism when Injected with Vaccinations
Tue May 8, 2012 11:18
174.233.134.32

Chapter Five, Update 1

Cure for AUTISM, UPDATE 1

For those who are new, we have published the "Cure" for about everything.

These "Cures" simply increase your immune system's ability to fight off the disease.

The process is simple:

1) Detoxify the body
2) Provide proper nutrients
3) Kill the bad bugs
4) Rebuild the good bugs - probiotics

Lots of extras help like Ed Skilling's Photon Genius, Hyperbaric Chambers, etc.

In this case we have been working with an 8 year Naval Veteran who is a Doctor. Her middle child is very autistic and is 8 years old - a little girl. She lives in her own world and has never interacted with another person - never.

One month of using Immusist and she actually spoke her first word. This is a literal Miracle. Here is what happened:

At school her teacher said "Good Morning Jan."

Jan waved back and said:" Good Morninnnn."

Then, after the school teacher points to Ariel she said: "Ariel."

Ariel spoke her first three words.

She connected a complicated word with a hand movement and then said a second word.

Over the last week she has learned to ride her bicycle alone - her hands and feet are now working together.

In addition - she came into the office and began interacting with the employees and playing and laughing with them - looking them in the eyes. She has never done that before.

When she says "I love you Mommy" we will immediately take the entire family out for dinner - on me.

Moms: Please see:
THE CAUSE OF AUTISM (Chapter 5, page 30)
THE CURE FOR CANCER, UPDATE 3 (Chapter 7, page 50)

The Veteran cried in my arms with joy as we both learned today she said her first words at 8 years old. She has only been using the Immusist for 1 month.

Total cost for this: The bottle cost about $110 and it will last her and her family 3 months.

If the AMA outlaws it we have 10 similar products to replace it.

One last thing - Cancer Survivors across the world are now reading these articles and posting them at cancer rallies. No one knows who is posting them - and since my name is on the article they refocus on me.

Chapter Five, Update 2

Cure for AUTISM, UPDATE 2

For those who are new:

We have been working with a doctor whose 8 year old child is autistic. In 8 years - not one word. This doctor did everything the "Medical Community" can do.

Along comes Dr. Mount:

After 30 days the child said two words;

1) Good Morn, waving her hand
2) Ariel, and then pointing.

The child was able to coordinate hand and mouth movement - a huge step.

The child was also interacting with people and riding a bicycle alone for the first time.

After 60 days:

1) The child said: Mommy.

2) The child is reciting the alphabet - 4 letters at a time. Personal Interaction has increased tremendously.

This is incredible - a Miracle.

When the child says: "Mommy, I love you": we go out and celebrate - no matter what time of day or night.

From a speechless child who never looked anyone in the eyes and was always in their own world then to a child actively interacting with folks, now connecting 4 words together and riding a bicycle in just 60 days.

This is repeated in child after child - Wow.

These reactions mentioned above are quite normal.

Chapter Five, Update 3

Cure for AUTISM, UPDATE 3

For those who have been following APFN you know we have been publishing the cure for a lot of diseases.

The Initial "The Cure for Cancer, Update 3" was published for Ben Fulford and for the Japanese people after Fukushima. He works hard, is pleasant to talk to, and is really trying to stabilize the world markets.

Please read the earlier stories:

THE CAUSE OF AUTISM (Chapter 5, page 30)
THE CURE FOR AUTISM, UPDATE 1 (Chapter 5-1, page 35)
THE CURE FOR AUTISM, UPDATE 2 (Chapter 5-2, page 38)

As you recall, about 6 months ago I walked into a Doctor's Office and 4 of the 9 people had cancer.

As we were walking three of the four out of cancer, the primary doctor shared with us that her 8 year old was Autistic.

Fast forward 3 months to today and we see some amazing things.

First, she is putting words together at an amazing rate.

Second, she is in information overload - she is going from 1 to 8 in 2 months and her little brain is overloaded. So - we slowed down a bit.

Third, her body is in toxic - overload. She is expelling all those toxins found in her vaccinations. She is physically sick from too many toxins. They will pass though.

Fourth - since she is on information overload - she cries a lot at night. She is afraid and over loaded so she cries. These symptoms are normal.

Fifth - we have been sprayed very heavily from jets lately. Chemical Trails are everywhere. Every autistic child in the area is sick - and I have a mild fever as well. The US Air Force out of Omaha is purposely making us sick and there is nothing we can do about it but pray GOD knocks them out of the sky ASAP.

Sixth - her head feels like it wants to explode at times. His neurons are reconnecting at a very rapid rate.

Seventh - the Husband refuses to participate. This may be more common than you think.

The Mom reassures her child that this is normal. She holds her a lot and for the first time the little girl understands and she can actually respond using 2 or 3 words at a time while using hand movement in conjunction with her speech.

This is normal - two steps forward and then you wait.

The only product the child has been using is Immusist.

See: Immusist.com

For those who have autistic children: It is about a 2 year road and the cost is about $100/month Total. It will be 5 years before they adjust to their new surroundings.

Just be patient and loving and realize each child responds differently to each set of stimuli and as you walk them out of Autism there will be some social skill problems - that's normal.

The Vaccinations really took their toll on these children.

What is exciting is to see a non-speaking child all glassy eyed now in a regular high school 7 years later with a 3.9 GPA.

What is also exciting is to watch the other kids in the family watch in utter amazement.

As a side note: Over the last few days I have come across the following documents:

1) Vaccination Compensation Table.

The primary reason for compensation after a vaccination is if it kills you. These vaccinations do such things as; stop your heart, swell up your air pipe and strangle you to death, shut down your brain, may cause a severe allergic reaction that leads to death - on and on it goes.

2) 42 USC 300aa-26 deals with vaccinations.

3) A flyer called: "Activated Influenza Vaccine 2011-12"

See: Immunize.org/vis

Symptoms from Vaccination: Fever, Sore Throat, Muscle Aches, Fatigue, Cough, Headache, Runny nose, DEATH.

Further - it discusses "Attenuated Vaccines: Live Virus.

Another thing discussed is that Guillain-Barre Syndrome (GBS) is not necessarily linked to Vaccinations... but if you read the literature the only people who got GBS were given vaccinations and there is no GBS found outside vaccinations. GBS - is crippling and then kills you.

In essence: Vaccinations contain things that make your child sick, autistic or dead.

The National Vaccination Compensation Program was started in 1986 and can be contacted by calling 1-800-338-2382 Free

1-800-338-2382. Remember - they are funded by Pig Pharma - do NOT trust them.

Pray that these folks with Autism read this and that GOD gives them the wisdom to walk their children out of Autism Immediately.

Chapter Five, Update 4

Cure for AUTISM, UPDATE 4

As you recall in previous stories Dr. ABC has an 8 year old child who WAS so autistic she never spoke or interacted with people.

We have been detoxifying her for three months and here are the results:

1) 30 Days: Said 2 words, interacting with people, riding a bicycle on her own.

2) 60 Days: Saying 5 letters in the Alphabet. Information overload and Toxicity Over Load. The daughter was sick from the USAF $9^{th}/10^{th}$ Air Wing in Omaha spraying the area with chemicals - or whatever the Air Wing calls itself now out of Omaha.

3) 90 Days: Now she is breaking out for the shell and is well and connecting the word "RED" with the color red, "Yellow" with yellow, etc. She knows all the colors - it is all locked up in her brain and now it is slowly surfacing.

Mentally she is growing about 4 times the rate of normal - emotionally? What we are seeing is that once the detoxification begins the Mental Age begins to progress.

In the case of those already in High School they seem to mentally grow enormously and emotionally grow at a normal rate.

Emotional Progression goes from age 0 to age 18.

If an autistic child begins detoxifying at age 10 then they will grow emotionally for 8 years until they are 18 years old.

You will have an 8 year old on your hands for life.

Thus the future adult stays as a child emotionally but may be in a clearer sense a child/genius for life.

Another 8 year old that was detoxified the old way began speaking at 10. He is now 15 and acts as a 5-6 year old. At maturity he will be 8-9years old for life, but smarter than any one of us.

What a Great Joy for Moms and Dads to watch this miracle occur to their own children and what a great joy it is to be part of this. The love that is sent out is over- whelming sometimes.

What happiness it is for mothers to know they are not failures. They now have Normal Kids, capable of not only receiving Love but of giving it.

Most Moms realize that most severely Autistic Children must be institutionalized during puberty costing the State about $300,000/ yr./child.

These techniques not only save the states Billions of Dollars but preserve the family and allow the child the opportunity to work.

A good profession for these Child Geniuses may be accounting or history teachers. These careers require smart folks.

There is hope for your Autistic Child and for your whole family.

You are NOT failures as parents, GOD did not make your child Autistic - we did. Now YOU can try steps to reverse it.

Friday I ran into a local Nurse at Cabela's Sporting Goods who told ME about this story. Her father was also in Hiroshima and knew about the Sea Weed to cure radiation sickness and cancer.

WOW - it's a small world.

Please see:

THE CURE FOR CANCER, UPDATE 3 (Chapter 7, page 50)
THE CURE FOR AUTISM, (Chapter 5, page 30-47)

Chapter Six

Cure for BURNS

Today we will discuss how to "Cure" burns.

If you are burned - blistered, house fire, stove burn just call this number as soon as you can - the faster the better:
...............818-332-6445..................

Keep it on your refrigerator; program it into your phone.

Already over 500 burn cases have been reported from over 32 countries.

1) My Personal Story: About 9 months ago I was burned on the stove. My finger blistered terribly. It hurt worse than a broken bone or being stabbed.

My wife brought me vanilla and it sort of helped.

Then I remembered the Burn Doctor.

I called 1-818-332-6446 FREE 1-818-332-6446 and reported it and within 5 minutes the pain went away.

The healing was remarkably fast - and no infection, and very little pain.

I am sorry I waited for an hour before calling.

There is no charge.

Exactly what they do - I am not sure - but it works and it is free.

2) A Little Girl's Story in Ghana - Adelaide: On 6 August 2010 little Adelaide's house caught on fire. Little Adelaide and her brother and sister were burned very badly. Little Adelaide was burned very badly. See the pictures on fireburndoctor.com.

A local Assemblyman in Ghana called the Fire Burn Doctor on the International Line (001-818-332-6445 FREE 001-818-332-6445) to ask for help for the burned children. The children were treated with the remote FBD method.

Little Adelaide (and her brother and sister) is now fine and shows very little scarring from her horrible burns. She is so happy to not have scars all over her little body.

You can see her pictures on Fireburndoctor.com.

So - keep that number handy for when you burn yourself next.

So Remember Moms and Dads: 1-818-332-6445.

Chapter Seven

Cure for CANCER, UPDATE 3

This is update #3 on the cure for cancer. This article will literally cover the cure for about anything that ails you - form Cancer to Lupus, from Diabetes to Lyme's Disease.

So here goes:

1) First you must decide to live. Whatever your ailment you must decide that the modern medical community got you here - sick - so let us look outside the "American Medical Box."

2) Begin with vitamins. We recommend you use Centrum Silver. Kelp is much better and if you can afford it buy it.

I personally found in me that Osteoporosis went away in 3 months, bone mass went from 65% - 105% in 3 months by using 1 Centrum every other day. VA records as shown on Ch 23 and 77 in Seattle.

3) Clean out your Liver and Kidneys with a tea of Burdock Root and Rose Hips. One teaspoon of each per week should do you.

4) To cure cancers add iodine.

We use one water purification tablet every other day - 8MG every other day. If you can afford Kelp Tablets instead - all the better.

1 Teaspoon of Kelp has 1.25MG iodine, you need 3 per day.

If you are allergic to Iodine clean out your system with the Ion Cleanse from E-bay for $120.

The "Cure" rate for the use of vitamins and Iodine is 97% over 10 years. Try that on for size and see how it fits.

In Chernobyl the Russian Government Workers were fed Potassium Iodide and were all dead within 2 years.

My adopted family in Kiev shoveled Radioactive Charcoal. After they were fed Miso Soup and Sea Weed they are alive today to talk about it.

When the U.S Army went into Hiroshima and Nagasaki just after the end of WW2 we discovered that those Japanese that moved back into the cities just after the blast that ate Miso Soup and Kelp lived, those that did not dies.

We used this method on my wife and here are the results: Cancer Tumors and Melanoma stopped growing in 6 weeks, the Melanoma and Tumors were gone in 6 months --- no scarring.

5) So what about Malaria (Parasite): Make a tea of the following ingredients all of equal parts - use 1 /2 teaspoon per day: Burdock

Root, Marshmallow, Dandelion Root, Rose Hips, Cloves, Bitter Wormwood (Artemisia Annua).

6) Plaque Build Up and high Blood Pressure: We use 1,000MG EDTA once per week only. Within 1 year my wife's blood pressure went down 35 points.

7) Age Extension: We are currently trying Blue Green Algae from Klamath Lake. The manufacturers claim it extends Human Life, got sued by the FDA and won - so - we are trying it.

8) Full Body Cleanse. The Ion Cleanse is found on EBay for about $120. It will help detoxify your body and according to many extends Human Life by 7 times. This machine is essential - buy lots of extra coils.

Remember - It takes 6 months to see real results so be patient.

ALTERNATIVE METHODS

1) Cancer: Many report the use of 1 Teaspoon of ***Baking Soda*** per day makes the body basic and the **Tumors stop right now.**

2) ***Turmeric***: This little spice not only stops tumor growth but reduces swelling and thus reduces your chances for a heart attack In fact - **prolonged use softens your veins and arteries and Plaque slowly comes off.** No more strokes, heart attacks, Aneurysms go down because blood pressure goes down, and cancer simply stops growing.

We use this daily on everything. We can afford it.

3) ***Citricare*** from Vim and Vigor: This is Glycerin Based citrus seed extract. The results against Fungal Infections (Including Cancer) are off the charts.

4) ***Hyperbaric Chambers***. The claims here are remarkable - everything from Lyme disease to Cancer is reduced to almost Zero, giving your body time to rest and recover.

Cost for a treatment runs about $100. The actual Hyperbaric Chamber runs around $10,000 a piece.

5) The ***Skilling*** Institute. The cells of each disease explode at a particular frequency. Ed has mapped the frequencies of so many diseases and added them to one single machine. Walk in with Cancer of Malaria - walk out Cancer or Malaria free.

The ***Photon Genius*** runs about $16,000 and every hospital should have one.

The portable Photon Genie runs about $3,500.

The other thing Ed has programmed into this machine are frequencies to stimulate you own cells - so you feel invigorated.

Imagine if a hospital had this machine - No more Malaria, Lyme disease, Cancer, etc.

6) ***Surfactants***. We have been using these gems for a while and the results are beyond belief.

a) ***Citricare*** uses Glycerin and gets rid of so many diseases including HIV - but it tastes horrible. When my wife or I get sick we reach for the bottle and use 100 drops and are fine the next day. It also is extremely effective as a Water Purifier - better than Iodine.

b) ***Immusist.*** This is a combination of 80 different Surfactants that are beneficial to Humans. I have been told by those involved incredible stories that I am personally finding true: Diabetes reversed in 2 months, Stage 4 Lung Cancer gone in 4 weeks; Autistic Children can speak in 12 months, in High School in 3 years. More will be mentioned on this product later.

I have even been told by an individual that his plaque in his veins and arteries are gone, and so is his Black Longs for 54 years of heavy smoking. WOW!

He said those 54 years of tar in his lungs - gone. No emphysema, no Asthma, no wheezing in 6 months of using Immusist.

The blood test on a child that could not speak - and the mom was told there was nothing the Medical Community could do for him - speaking in 12 months; his eyes were no longer glazed over. Hundreds of moms tell the same story over and over again.

Military Moms with deformed children by the dozens - their children complete idiots - now in school - normal schools.

If I had no money I would buy Immusist and **Kelp**.

Wow - when a Mom sees her child able to speak for the first time in 10 years - watch out. She will tell the world, and this is just what is happening. You can't take away a mom's license to speak out, can you?

I bind those who are to come against the techniques and Companies in this article and I turn you over to the destruction of your flesh and I command the demons in these people to the Fiery Pit for all eternity, in the name of the King of Kings and Lord of Lords, who was and is and is to come, and in the name of HIS son Jeshua.

Time and experience is a better teacher than anything.

Oh, yes - we have great degrees that hanging on the wall, certificates abound - but there is nothing like the school of Hard Knocks.

I have a friend (Let's call him Jeff) who came to me about 2 months ago with a "Pre-Cancerous" Growth. It was a sort of wart in a rather odd place. I gave him the website of: THE CURE FOR CANCER, UPDATE 3 (and Chapter 7, page 50).

Well - Jeff was so happy he went to a Naturopath Doctor, who proceeded to give him Iodine Trichloride.

Iodine Trichloride is a very deadly poison and does not allow your body to use the Iodine. The theory here is to displace the Chlorine, Bromine and Fluorine with Iodine. Now how does that happen with 1 Iodine and three (Tri) chlorine? Besides the Material Data Safety Sheet lists these as Poison.

After 3 months his cancer is still there - unchanged.

Jeff is no slouch - his income dwarfs mine and he is extremely intelligent.

So we went right to my home and I read him. He has been smoking a little "Green" stuff (Legal here in Washington) and he had lung cancer. The Warts he was growing were just a reflection of the part of his body that had cancer.

There is a range in the middle of his lungs that are beginning to turn black.

So does this not disprove the idea that Dope cures Cancer?

So I gave him some:

1) Turmeric - it stops the Growth of the Tumors Right Now!
2) Water Purification Tablets - Iodine.
3) Citricare - to knock back his Yeast Infection.
4) Centrum Silver Vitamins.
5) Immusist - to clean out his lungs.
6) EDTA - to clean out the blocked veins and arteries he now has. Yes - Turmeric does this too, just not as fast.

Two days later he called me. He has been rubbing the warts with Immusist and they are going away.

Within 6 months his cancer will be totally gone.

Total Cost to remove cancer in 6 months:

1) Turmeric: 1 Bottle per month: $45.
2) Water Purification Tablets, 2 bottles: $20.
3) Citricare, 1 Bottle: $36.
4) Centrum Silver, 1 Bottle: $14
4) Immusist: 2 Bottles: $180.
6) EDTA, 1 Bottle: $20.

Total Cost over 6 months: About $335, or about $55 per month.

His whole attitude is so completely different about life now.

He did not have cancer - he had a Nutrient Deficiency.

What you do with YOUR life is between YOU and GOD.

Please Pray that you come to terms with YOUR diseases and take these "Cures" seriously.

Chapter Eight

Cure for CEREBRAL PALSY

The theory is that this Hyperbaric Chamber combined with an Oxygen Generator forces oxygen into the cells, kicking out diseases.

The Chamber takes you down to the equivalent 11 feet under water - that's all - but wow - what a rush - like a great cup of coffee for the rest of your life naturally.

So what else is it good for:

There is a gal in my home town that was in a wheel chair and was told by her doctors to get some diapers because it is downhill from here. She went to 2 treatments per week and after 6 weeks was walking full time without a wheel chair.

Swelling: Many Ambulances in Japan have these chambers as part of their normal treatment. This forces air into a wound and this reduces swelling and secondary injury caused by swelling.

Many folks use the chamber before an operation to reduce swelling after the operation.

Cerebral Palsy: There have been improvements after three treatments. The local folks are still testing but results look good. The problem is - most CP patients do not have enough money to do 40 treatments and Medicare will not cover this machine - even though others who treat CP patients say it cures them. Apparently $4,000 is too much to put a person back to work.

They need to rethink their policy - the State and Feds need to treat people and make them well rather than string them along with drugs until they die.

Treatment runs about $100 for a one hour session. We used the Vitaeris 320 with the Oxygen Generator. Total cost for the unit is around $28,000.

Consider the alternative!

If you need a small portable unit you can purchase the Solace for about $12,000.

Russia: How much better would your Olympic Athletes do if you had the 4 or 5 full scale Vitaeris Chambers with an Oxygen Generator for your athletes?

No more Silver Medals, all Gold.

Many people sleep in these chambers. Tests show that after 40 treatments (2x/wk.) Adult Stem Cell Count is up 800%. Imagine how fast your athletes would heal if you used this chamber.

Many believe the increase in Stem Cells stops the aging process - time will tell. Either way - 12 hours later I still feel great.

You may purchase these at H3 Therapy at: 253-432-0022 FREE 253-432-0022.

Or Bill at: 253-857-3220 FREE 253-857-3220 or 253-509-8552 FREE 253-509-8552.

I hold no financial interest in any corporation, the FBI made sure of that when we put Russian Troops in Iran and seized 300 Nukes built by the USA for the Shaw of Iran and stopped the US/Iranian war in 2007.

When I recommend companies I do so because I believe in them and their products.

Chapter Nine

Cure for DIABETES

First follow the protocols of the Cure for Cancer, Update 3 (Chapter 7, page 50). Consider adding Citricare and Immusist to your daily regimen.

But above all keep your body Alkaline = NON ACIDIC the use of a teaspoon of Baking Soda mixed in a glass of water will assist you in making your body alkaline. The theory is that this Hyperbaric Chamber combined with an Oxygen Generator forces oxygen into the cells, kicking out diseases.

The Chamber takes you down to approximately 11 feet under water - that's all - but wow - what a rush - like a great cup of coffee for the rest of your life naturally.

Swelling: Many Ambulances in Japan have these chambers as part of their normal treatment. This forces air into a wound thus reducing swelling and secondary injury caused due to swelling. Many folks use the chamber before an operation to reduce swelling after the operation.

Apparently $4,000 is too much to put a person back to work. They need to rethink their policy - the State and Feds need to treat people and make them well rather than string them along with drugs until they die.

Diabetes, the Literature is full of personal stories of how this amazing product works.

Treatment runs about $100 for a one hour session. We used the Vitaeris 320 with the Oxygen Generator. Total cost for the unit is around $28,000.

Consider the alternative!

If you need a small portable unit you can purchase the Solace for about $12,000.

Many people sleep in these chambers. Tests show that after 40 treatments (2X/Wk) Adult Stem Cell Count is up 800%. Imagine how fast you would heal if you used this chamber.

Many believe the increase in Stem Cells stops the aging process - time will tell. Either way - 12 hours later I still feel great.

You may purchase these at H3 Therapy at: 253-432-0022 FREE 253-432-0022.

Or Bill at: 253-857-3220 FREE 253-857-3220 or 253-509-8552 FREE 253-509-8552.

I hold no financial interest in any corporation, the FBI made sure of that when we put Russian Troops in Iran and seized 300 Nukes built by the USA for the Shaw of Iran and stopped the US/Iranian war in 2007.

When I recommend companies I do so because I believe in them and their products.

Chapter Ten

Cure for DEPLETED URANIUM

Radiation Damage: Many feel that the Hyperbaric Chamber is the only way to heal tissue damaged by radiation. See also Cure for Cancer, Update 3 (Chapter 7, page 50).

Chapter Eleven

Cure for GULF WAR SYNDROME

Ed Skilling Photon Genie runs about $3000 and kills all affected cells in your body.

Hyperbaric Chamber - this is very effective. They run around $24,000 but do so much more for your body.

Citricare from Vim and Vigor: This runs about $40 shipped to you and knocks back the HIV virus into infinity. They make no claims about this - but I do.

I wish I had a million bottles of this to give to our dying troops who came back from the First Gulf War. Many were given the HIV Virus - see the Senate and Congressional Reports we talked about last night on APFN for verification.

Over 100,000 of the 660,000 Gulf War ground Troops were Dying or dead within 2 years of coming home.

Immusist: Try it. Go to Immusist.com. Read the testimonies. Cost: $100 shipped. Just do it.

Turmeric: Just use it - it reduces inflammation.

As in all "Cures" you need a vitamin base - I recommend starting with Centrum Silver every other day.

If you can afford it - use 5 -10 Kelp Tablets a day instead of Centrum. The added minerals will keep you from getting HIV Associated Cancer.

By the way - we in the U.S. Army have had the cure for it since before it was released. Now you know - we have gone public. It was in our U.S. Army Field Manuals before the First Gulf War.

After the First Gulf War most references to Nuclear/Chemical and Bio weapons were burned. Even President Ronald Regan's First Army Film as a Second Lieutenant - a film on Foot care - was burned.

Remember - HIV can lay dormant in your cells for years so keep this stuff around just in case it comes back. No disease is ever really CURED, just knocked back long enough to let your immune system recover.

See Also: CURE FOR CANCER, UPDATE 3 (Chapter 7, page 50)

Pray - Visualize p- that you go down a path that leads you to being healthy - whatever path is right for you.

CHAPTER TWELVE

Cure for HEART DISEASE

We hear allot of things on TV and the Radio about Heart disease - but what exactly is it, how do we get it and most importantly - how do we get rid of it?

Well - here we go:

1) What is Heart Disease? Well - you're Veins and Arteries become brittle. When they swell due to Food Additives, GMOs, exercise they crack.

The Cracks are then filled with Plaque and then calcify over and your blood vessels become clogged, your Blood Pressure rises, and often times your Blood Vessels swell and you get an Aneurysm.

If you experience additional swelling around the heart your heart stops.

If your Aneurysm busts open you usually bleed to death - yuck.

Twelve years ago my own heart stopped while I was playing a Guitar. I reached down and - no pulse. Everything slowed down like in

"Saving Private Ryan." I asked GOD what HE wants me to do and my Right Hand formed a fist and smacked 'em in my chest and everything returned to normal. Shortly after this I found myself on another journey. I was only 42 at the time.

It can strike at any age.

2) What causes Heart Disease: We all know this. It is too much fat and Sugar, too little exercise, food additives, water additives, and overall poor health habits.

3) How do we cure Heart Disease: This is so easy.

First - I recommend 1 Centrum Silver 3 times per week as a bases for all treatments.

a) The easiest way is to eat lots of Grass Fed Meet - like Pork, beef, deer, moose, and elk. The owner of Skagit Valley Farms had a Quadruple Bypass and joined the "Zipper Club" many years ago. He started his own farm up Highway 2 (North of Seattle) and within one year of eating his own Butter, Lard, Beef and Chicken he had plaque buildup - it was all gone.

The Organic Grass Fed meat is really good also.

b) For you Vegetabletarians - EDTA. I use 1,200 MG once per week and within 1 year ALL of my plaque buildup was gone and my veins were soft again so as they swell they do not crack any more. My Blood Pressure is usually 120 over 70.

Start SLOW. Start with One tablet per week and work up to 6 or 6 tablets per week over a month period.

c) Turmeric. This little Gem of a Spice eliminates swelling so no more Heart Attacks. Wives - use this in everything you cook and you and your Husband's Blood Vessels will remain flexible and young. Unfortunately it does not cure wrinkles.

d) Surfactant. Soap (Surfactant) cleans out Cholesterol. Again - start with only 1-43 drops per day. Two products I have used are:

A) Citricare from Vim and Vigor. Put this in Fruit Juice and use a pinch of Baking Soda - you cannot taste the stuff.

B) Immusist.com is Very Very effective.

e) Ed Skilling's Machine

There are frequencies for dissolving Kidney Stones, Plaque and rejuvenating the cells.

If you have $3,000 buy the Photon Genie - you will not be sorry.

Warren - who runs Ed's Lab right now - is one remarkable man. Ed's Research never ends so the machine just gets better and better.

If you are completely broke - just buy Centrum Silver, Turmeric and when you can get it - EDTA. The total cost here is about $40 and it will last you an entire year.

As in all "Cures" we just reverse the Course of the Disease but one must make a Life Style Change to keep these diseases at bay.

I think lowering my wife's blood pressure by 40 points and eliminating her Cancer and her heart arrhythmia in one year is a pretty good sign we are on the right track, don't you?

By the way - I have no financial interest in any of the companies I have mentioned - in fact; thanks to the FBI I have no stocks at all.

I tell you about them because I currently use their product. It took me many years to find these products and counter the Nuclear/ Chemical/ Biological weapons I was exposed to and it is an ongoing process.

So here are the ways to eliminate Heart Disease once and for all:

1) EDTA - my Favorite. I use 1000MG once per week,. That is all you need. After 1 year I had no plaque in my Arteries of Veins and they are very Flexible. You can buy it on line or at a Natural Health Food Store.

2) My second Favorite: Organic Grass Fed Beef. The Owner of Skagit Valley Farms had a Quadruple Bypass - I mean it likes spaghetti around his heart. After the operation he and his wife decided to start a farm. After one year of eating grass fed beef he had NO plaque buildup in his veins and arteries - and they were flexible.

Remember - Grass Fed *only*, no grain.

3) Fish oil. I have not used this but have read that there is limited success in removing Plaque from your Arteries and Veins.

4) Ground Up Roughage. There is an internet Rumor that ground up Avocado Pits remove plaque. I tried it - yuck. We do know that the higher the roughage in a diet the lower the plaque builds up.

5) Exercise. When I was running I had now Plaques build up at all. When I stopped running due to an Army Injury the Plaque in my Arteries and Veins built up fast. You will need about 30 minutes of Hard Exercise every other day to keep you from clogging up.

6) Surfactants. Yup - human digested surfactants clean you out slick as a whistle. We are currently using 2:
   a) Immusist. This is very very effective and at about $108 for a bottle very affordable. A bottle lasts around 3 months.
   b) Citricare from Vim and Vigor.

7) Dr Ed Skilling of The Skilling Institute has had great success in cleaning out your arteries and veins.

What do I do?

I use the EDTA, Immusist, and Citricare and I eat Skagit Valley Beef because I happen to really like the owner.

When I can afford to buy Ed Skilling's Machine I will.

Please see: APFN THE CURE FOR CANCER, UPDATE 3 (Chapter 7, page 50)

The Cure for Cancer is dedicated to Lita Marshal, who died a month before I discovered the cure, the wife of a very good friend.

El Rushbo - this Cure for Heart Disease (Chapter 12, page 67) is dedicated to you because you had the guts to speak the truth about Heart Disease.

Chapter Thirteen

Cure for HIV

CURE FOR HIV

1) What is HIV

Way back in the early 1960's the US Department of Agriculture, in conjunction with the Plum Island U.S. Army Bio Weapons Program, went to Montana and collected samples of Sheep Wasting Disease. It was brought back to the lab and grown.

This bug is what we refer to as a "Super Virus."

2) How did it get released?

During the Metal Wars of the 1970's the Russians placed a "Ring of War" around Rhodesia and South Africa. This forced Millions of Blacks to move into these nations. This overload of population was meant to over stress their economic systems and force the closing of Chrome Mines in these countries.

South Africa responded by mining their northern border - but too many Elephants were blown up on the northern border so, due to international pressure, the mining ended.

In response the US sent Hepatitis B vaccinations to give to the population around the Rothschild's Chrome and Diamond Mines laced with HIV.

Rhodesia was invaded by Cuba, they came back and sent their Sick Gay Troops (Being GAY is illegal in Cuba) who got HIV in Rhodesia to Miami, New York and San Francisco.

For many years in the Intel Community it was a joke: AIDS is not working fast enough to kill off the liberals.

3) How can I get HIV:

First - sex with another HIV carrier. Condoms do no good in preventing the spread of HIV.

Second - Mosquito or tick bite. It a Mosquito bites an HIV carrier and bite you then you have a 5% chance of getting HIV. This was determined in an internal U.S. Army Study. It is available on the VA restricted Archives to VA doctors and nurses only.

Third - Blood Transfusion

Fourth - A Kiss. Yes - a kiss can spread all sorts of VD, including HIV. Think about it.

4) So how do I get rid of this horrible HIV?
Remember - Magic Johnson *announced* he had AIDS way back in 1991, and he is still alive after 21 years.

First - see your doctor and treat yourself for all the other diseases you have picked up.

Second - there are several products that eliminate HIV. If the FDA or a state outlaws them there are 100 waiting in the wings. I will simply republish this article. These products are:

a) Ed Skilling Photon Genie. It runs about $3000 and kills all HIV cells in your body.

b) Hyperbaric Chamber - this is very effective. They run around $24,000 but do so much more for your body.

Third - Citricare from Vim and Vigor. This runs about $40 shipped to you and knocks back the HIV virus into infinity. They make no claims about this - but I do.

I wish I had a million bottles of this to give to our dying troops who came back from the First Gulf War. Many were given the HIV Virus - see the Senate and Congressional Reports we talked about last night on APFN for verification.

Over 100,000 of the 660,000 Gulf War ground Troops were Dying or dead within 2 years of coming home.

Fourth - Immusist. Try it. Go to Immusist.com. Read the testimonies. Cost: $100 shipped. Just do it.

Fifth - Turmeric. Just use it - it reduces inflammation.

As in all "Cures" you need a vitamin base - I recommend starting with Centrum Silver every other day.

If you can afford it - use 5 -10 Kelp Tablets a day instead of Centrum. The added minerals will keep you from getting HIV Associated Cancer.

By the way - we in the U.S. Army have had the cure for HIV/AIDS since before it was released. Now you know - we have gone public. It was in our U.S. Army Field Manuals before the First Gulf War.

After the First Gulf War most references to Nuclear/Chemical and Bio weapons were burned. Even President Ronald Regan's First Army Film as a Second Lieutenant - a film on Foot care - was burned.

Remember - HIV can lay dormant in your cells for years so keep this stuff around just in case it comes back. No disease is ever really CURED, just knocked back long enough to let your immune system recover.

The Cure for HIV was published in Honor of Michigan Governor Snyder and Michigan Senator Randy Richardville for purposely destroying the small farmers in Michigan.

This article would not have been published without them - so call them and thank them.

Thank you for reading the: SNYDER/RICHARDVILLE CURE FOR AIDS.

See Also: CURE FOR CANCER, UPDATE 3 (Chapter 7, page 50)

Pray - Visualize p- that you go sown a path that leads you to being healthy - whatever path is right for you.

Chapter Fourteen

The Cure for LYME DISEASE

A MESSAGE TO THE LYME COMMUNITY

As in all cases - the "Cures" we talk about are about 90-97% effective and allow the body time to heal so it can overcome the disease.

Lyme disease is one of 254 types (As of the year 1995) of Relapsing Fevers.

It was first cloned way back in 1994 in the U.S. Army Bio Weapons Factory in Plum Island New York and began infecting folks in New York soon after wards. It got loose - right through the air filtration system. It was a Bio Weapon - Oops! Captain - Biological Warfare - me, remember?

Eventually the Disease worked its way north into Lyme Connecticut where a Doctor differentiated it from the other 253 forms of Relapsing Fever.

There are 2 different forms of Relapsing Fevers that show the distinct Round Rash around the tick bite, only one of them is Lyme disease. Both are deadly.

One big problem with Lyme Disease it that the U.S. Army Purposely injected Lyme Patients with Malaria and other diseases to counter the Lyme Disease - I still have the original copy of the study.

So a typical Lyme disease Patient has usually also contracted Malaria, Rocky Mountain Spotted Fever, Microplasma Ferensis Incognitos and many other diseases - as it was in my case.

When you treat yourself be very careful - your immune system is shot.

1) Use the tetracycline the doctor gives you. In an emergency these antibiotics may be found in a feed store - be very careful.

2) Use Citricare to counter the negative effects of antibiotics. Vim and Vigor makes Citricare.

3) Use a tea to clean out your liver, kidneys and kill parasites like Malaria of equal parts of:
   Burdock Root
   Marshmallow
   Rose Hops
   Dandelion Root
   Bitter Wormwood (Artemisia Annua) - Used for Malaria in 190 countries.
   Cloves - kills Parasite eggs, great for flavor also.

4) Cleanse yourself with the Ion Cleanse, eBay, $120.

5) Immusist.com - although only now being tested on Lyme disease is 100% effective on ALL diseases it was tested on.

6) Buy Ed Skilling's Photon Genie for $3,500 - it actually blows the Lyme Cells apart. The problem is Lyme hides - so you will need to use and reuse it.

7) Hyperbaric Chamber with Oxygen Therapy - there are films available that shows Lyme Disease Cells spiraling out of Red Blood Cells when in a Chamber and using Oxygen.

8) As in all cases: Either use one Centrum Silver 4 times a week or use 3 Kelp Tablets daily.

9) Your gut bacteria is toast - use Probiotics. I started with Bifa 15 from Edan Foods.

10) If you are a veteran and cannot work - go to the VA immediately and apply for the Veteran's Pension - it is $1000+ per month and at least it will feed you and house you and buy some of these basic products for you.

It is a long slow recovery because of the damage these diseases do to your Human Body - but you WILL recover.

The unfortunate part is Lyme Disease (Relapsing Fever) Keeps on Relapsing.

The idea is to control it enough to live a more normal life. I know what it is to be in bed with Lyme Disease for months while doctors tell you it is all *mental.* I know what it feels like to be crippled from this disease for years. It is the most horrible feeling in the world.

After months in bed I was actually retired from the U.S. Army from the "Results of Lyme Disease." The damage to my heart from Lyme and the other diseases still haunts me - but I whipped it fair and square and rarely get fevers any more.

Cured - well, able to keep it well under control - how is that?

Just remember - there is hope.

THE CURE FOR CANCER, UPDATE 3 (Chapter 7, page 50).

When Update 3 is erased by the Cyber NAZI's (U.S. Army Cyber Command) - then will publish Update 4.

I have full Diplomatic Immunity and Royal Prerogative to continue helping you out and will continue to publish as long as possible.

You have RIGHT to get well - and to know your options.

This is meant as a resource guide to point you in the right direction.

Find out what works for YOU and then use it.

A MESSAGE TO THE LYME COMMUNITY

To the Lyme Community:

In 1992 I was exposed to Lyme Disease as well as Ehrlichiosis, Babesiosis, Malaria, Microplamsa Incognetis, and a host of other diseases while on Active Duty in the U.S. Army as a young Second Lieutenant.

These diseases were cloned in Plum Island, New York and were designer bio weapons created to kill us. For example: 70% of the Alzheimer's cases we find Lyme Disease in the brain.

I have seen what the NAZI FDA does to doctors who actually treat Lyme Patients. Now that we are under full Martial Law they can do darn near anything.

*The purpose of my article; Chapter APFN THE CURE FOR LYME DISEASE is to focus the FDA NAZIs on me, and to take the focus away from you.

With Full Diplomatic Immunity and Full Royal Prerogative as recognized by International Law I am the only "World Citizen" who has never broken the law or signed a "Non Disclosure Agreement." The last time the FBI NAZIs touched me the market fell from 14.2 to 6.9. A signal was sent to our U.S. NAZIs to leave me alone a few short months ago when 2 underground bases were destroyed - one in Mineral Virginia and one in Trinidad ---- remember the Washington, D.C. Earthquake that emanated from Mineral, Virginia?

It is not the Eastern Block that should scare the FDA NAZIs - but the Living GOD, the King of Kings and Lord of Lords and what HE will do to them if they touch me.

I slipped through the cracks as a World Citizen, all glory goes to the Living GOD.

At first I did not know what I was exposed to - it took me almost 6 years to discover this fact. I had to go to a very special Laboratory to do the testing - and this Doctors daughter was also dying from the Gulf War Crap.

I also had the opportunity to be exposed to those creating Bio Weapons. They are not ashamed of their work - cloning Sheep Wasting Disease into HIV, or Relapsing Fever into 254 different forms - only one of which is Lyme Disease. These folks work very hard to create these designer diseases. Too bad many get loose - oops!

I will never expose a doctor for treating any one, nor will I quote any of their articles. The FDA NAZIs are too underhanded and ruthless and the doctors have no recourse once confronted by these NAZIs.

Fortunately - these "Cures" are now published (And used) in India, China, Russia, etc. The first one being published about 5 months ago: APFN THE CURE FOR CANCER (Chapter 7, page 50). The Cat is Out of the bag. That is how far my articles travel in a day or two.

Those in the Eastern Block of Nations read these articles very carefully and after they confirm them usually take immediate action - including implementing these protocols in their nations.

Just remember Lyme Doctor's - you can always say: "I asked the patient to look at Dr. Mount's Treatment Regime."

For you Moms who have kids who are very sick - my present to you.

CURE FOR LYME DISEASE (Chapter 14, page 78).

Try Also: CURE FOR LYME DISEASE --- Note how US Cyber Command changed my original title to screw you up.

See Also: CURE FOR CANCER, UPDATE 3 (Chapter 7, page 50)

Chapter Fifteen

Cure for MALARIA

So what about Malaria (Parasite): Make a tea of the following ingredients all of equal parts - use 1 /2 teaspoon per day: Burdock Root, Marshmallow, Dandelion Root, Rose Hips, Cloves, Bitter Wormwood (Artemisia Annua).

See also: THE CURE FOR CANCER, UPDATE 3 (Chapter 7, page 50).

Chapter Sixteen

Cure for MUSCULAR DYSTROPHY (MS)

1) What is MS: MS, like HIV, they are an auto immune disease leaving you open to various infections and in the case of MS it affects your nerves in your backbone.

2) What causes MS: Toxicity! The over toxicity causes your immune system to fail and wham - a virus like Herpes eats the Myelin Sheath on your nerves and you have MS.

3) How do I get rid of MS: Here is the great part, in most cases it is "Reversible." You must detoxify your body and feed it nutrients. For every treatment I recommend we use 1 Centrum Silver Vitamin every other day - you can buy them anywhere. You can use Good Quality Kelp Pills at 2 per day, but this is more costly.

Here are the "Cures," way to reverse MS:::::

a) Ed Skilling's Photo Genie. The cost is about $3,600 but it stops MS in its tracks. Period. See Skilling Institute.

b) Immusist. Start Slowly - you have a lot of Toxins in your body. It will take several months to detoxify your body. So far tests show it is 100% effective. You will need about 1 bottle every 3 months. Cost: $33/mo. Go to Immusist.com.

c) The old tried and true. Use the Ion Cleanse on EBay - it runs $120 and you will use one coil per month. Use this in conjunction with Immusist and WOW - you detoxify fast. It runs about 50 cents to detox for 30 minutes.

Also: Do not forget to have on hand Citricare from Vim and Vigor. I use 100 drops when I get sick and the next day I am always fine.

Also: See CURE FOR CANCER, UPDATE 3 (7, page 46).

You have the right to be MS free.

When you are MS free share this with your doctor.

Before you begin any treatment ask GOD for HIS guidance. This is only a Guide Book and intended for your use.

When your MS begins to subside - do not thank me, thank the BIG GUY upstairs. I am only a messenger.

Cure for autism - Immusist, the Ion Cleanse, and Kelp.

1) First you must decide to live. Whatever your ailment you must decide that the modern medical community got you here - sick - so lets us look outside the "American Medical Box."

2 Begins with vitamins. We recommend you use Centrum Silver. Kelp is much better and if you can afford this use it.

I personally found in me that Osteoporosis went away in 3 months, bone mass went from 65% - 105% in 3 months by using 1 Centrum every other day. VA records as shown on Ch 23 and 77 in Seattle.

3) Clean out your Liver and Kidneys wit a tea of Burdock Root and Rose Hips. One teaspoon of each per week should do you.

4) To cure cancers just add iodine.

So here is the cure:

Type In: CURE FOR CANCER

Add the following to your daily tea:

1) Bitter Wormwood (Artemisia Annua) - Kills Parasites

2) Cloves - kills parasite eggs

Add Citricare from Vim and Vigor

Morgellons disease is a horrible disease where metal splinters poke through your skin - it hurts like the dickens.

The symptoms are identical to Mercury poisoning described 150 years ago.

So you got 2, 3, 5, 8...Vaccinations as a kid loaded with mercury and you eat fish loaded with mercury and you live near a coal fired power plant pumping mercury into the air and you wonder why you have Morgellons?

So how do you cure it?

Type into Google: APFN THE CURE FOR CANCER (Chapter 7, page 50)

CHAPTER SEVENTEEN

Cure for OSTEOPOROSIS

Begin with vitamins. We recommend you use Centrum Silver. Kelp is much better and if you can afford this then use it.

I personally found in me that Osteoporosis went away in 3 months, bone mass went from 65% - 105% in 3 months by using 1 Centrum every other day. VA records as shown on Ch 23 and 77 in Seattle.

Chapter Eighteen

Cure for PARKINSON DISEASE

Parkinson's disease is in one of the local Grocery Store Blats.

In this horrible disease part of your brain actually dies and your body's nervous system literally breaks down, similar to MS.

Parkinson's is degrading of your entire nervous system due to a Genetically Modified Epstein Virus - the same one used to give kids Autism.

Headaches can be severe and you get intense ones between the eyes which cause you to get dizzy.

Occasionally you have ringing in your ears.

To much rich food and not enough nutrition can be your downfall. Your doctor's plan on Chemo and Radiation - will kill you.

Here is what you do:

You will be using what is found in 3 articles:

THE CURE FOR CANCER, UPDATE 3 (Chapter 7, page 50)
THE CURE FOR HIV/Aides (Chapter 13, page 73)
THE CURE FOR HEART DISEASE (Chapter 12, page 67)

Chapter Nineteen

The 'CURE' for PTSD

This is perhaps the hardest thing to talk about.

When a Soldier is sent to war he usually comes back with memories that no person should have.

He wonders why he was sent there and what he was doing there.

The sights of dead burnt bodies and putting another person in your sights can be horrifying.

When my Father-In-Law was in WW2 he served on a large Slow Target (LST124). After the invasion of Saipan he could take no more. The rest of the war was spent repairing the ship and resupplying the other invasions.

For many years all he could talk about in Private Conversations was Saipan.

My father In Law just recently died and at 86 his last words were "12 Inches" He was referring to a Navy Joke he had heard in 1944 - 68 years ago.

He had the night mares, the night sweats, the anger outbursts, etc. You know what I mean.

When you sit down and relive these things your face actually becomes hot, your muscles tense up, and your eyes get pinpoint. You can actually see things from the past.

I have seen several soldiers in my command go into a "Flash-Back" and begin wondering through the woods as if they are somewhere else. I understand fully. Thank GOD none of them used drugs so as soon as we recognized it we contained them. I was able to walk them all into retirement.

So what the heck do you do about it?

1) Realize you are normal. Talk to others about it - this is normal to feel this way, *You* are not alone.

Many combat vets stay connected in the National Guard and Reserves so as to have a base of folks to talk to about their experiences.

2) Get involved.

Go to Veteransaid.com and check out what is available for you.

Get involved with the local AMVETS of DAV Chapters - volunteer.

GO hang with the AMVETS, or help with the American Legion - they love it. They like Volunteers.

Help fight to keep us out of Syria and Iran.

3) I urge you to stay away from Illegal Drugs and Alcohol. It will not make you forget.

4) Give it to GOD.

5) How I deal with PTSD: I fight.

I fight for Freedom, for America, for our veterans. I do not drink.

When I really get to feeling sorry for myself or see those who dies protecting me - I think about my promise to one soldier: "I Will Make It Better." and it drives me forward.

When I need Physical Work to slow me down I go outside and build a Chicken Coop or Barn. I keep Busy.

I feel good about the 2 Veteran's Cases I won this year, walking a child out of autism, publishing the APFN Cure for Cancer, Update 3 (and Chapter 7, page 50).

Then I get on my knees and ask GOD to forgive me for following, being forced to follow a bunch of lying politicians and doing what I did. I felt it was right at the time.

I am not Depressed (Repressed Anger) but angry at those who are creating this constant war. By expressing this, my Anger and Fear go away.

Fear leads to Anger, Anger leads to Hate, Hate leads to Depression.

Just Remember: "I did not start the war, the Rothschild's did and I am angry at them and GOD will now deal directly with them. I only answered to my nation's call."

I also play allot of Harp Praise GOD music. Any Harp will do.

Thunder Hawk Music also calms the Savage Soul.

Since I am retired I hang with the local Civil War Association - WCWA. One of the Battery Commander is a retired Command Sergeant Major and we talk allot. Our navy units are filled with Nam Vets and we can talk openly about how I feel and they have been there - so they can talk to me as well.

6) If it gets bad enough you may wish to go to a VA doctor - but remember: PTSD is a Psychological Disorder and once diagnosed you may lose your right to keep and bear arms - so do so as a last resort.

The VA hospitals now have great food courts and here in Tacoma do a pretty good job with our vets thanks to Marilyn Capize, the Legislative Representative. I have worked with her now for about 2 years and medical care has greatly improved here thanks to her.

Remember: A box of chocolates can open allot of doors at the VA Hospitals.

Chapter Twenty

Cure for TRAUMATIC BRAIN INJURY

This is dedicated to all our service members coming home with TBI.

The "Cure" means that put your body in a position for it to heal itself,. In this case - we have seen some real miracles with TBI.

A Traumatic brain Injury is usually caused by some sort of Trauma to the brain. Maybe you fall down in a Bicycle Accident, are injured in a Sport, or get near an Improvised Explosive Device (IED).

No matter what the cause - you brain is jostled and then injured.

Over 1.75 Million Americans received some sort of TBI every year, and around 175,000 are permanently injured.

For the Military this rate is extremely high due to Combat injuries such as explosions, hitting your head, etc.

Years ago in the Military I was near an explosion and afterwards I wondered aimlessly for about 5-10 Minutes before I could get my own bearings. The headache that remained was pretty intense. After handling explosives for many years as a Combat Engineer, this kind of injury was common.

In many cases - the injury does not appear to go away so the soldiers had to be evacuated to the rear.

So what do you do if you get a TBI:

1) Immediately: Treat for swelling to reduce the immediate injury.

In Japan about one half the Ambulances have Hyperbaric Chambers and on transport for a TBI they put the patient in the chamber to reduce swelling. It also seems to help control Internal Bleeding.

About 200 NFL Football Players have a Hyperbaric Chamber and use them to speed up their healing process. This is why a guy can break a leg and play 3 weeks later - he is completely healed. It is that good.

In America treatment for swelling does not occur until the patient is hospitalized, which is why so many TBI folk become disabled.

The best thing a Mom can do to prevent this kind of long term injury is: Add Turmeric to all of her cooking - ALL OF IT.

Put it on eggs, in Cereal, on sandwiches, etc. A family of 4 should go through at least 2 bottles per month. It is almost flavorless.

If your child is injured the Turmeric will prevent a large portion of the swelling and your child will receive less damage form a head injury.

I would also like to see Ed Skilling's Photon Genius mounted in each and every US Ambulance as it would boost the immune system and help reduce swelling, thus reducing long-term injury. The cost would be around $3,500 but would reduce long-term medical care of patients by literally billions.

Imagine the money Insurance companies would save with a Hyperbaric and Ed Skilling's Machine in every Ambulance?

2) What if the TBI was last week, or last year?

Follow the course set out in: APFN THE CURE FOR CANCER, UPDATE 3 (Chapter 7, page 50).

These are:

a) Detoxify

Use Immusist
Use Ion Cleanse found on E-bay
Try LDM-100. Be careful - powerful stuff. Start very slowly.

b) Nutrify

Use 6-10 Kelp Tablets per day

or

One Centrum Silver + 1 8MG Iodine Tablet 3 times per week. That gives you an average of 23.5MG Iodine/day. In Japan the average is 12.5MG/day - so this is way under and is generally a safe dose in my opinion.

We also add Vitamin A, C, and D-3 plus Blue Green Algae from Klamath Lake, Oregon 3X/Wk.

c) Kill the bad bugs

Use Citricare from Vim and Vigor
and
Use Immusist

Drink my tea 5X/wk of
Burdock Root
Rose Hips
Dandelion Root
Marshmallow
Artemisia Annua - Bitter Wormwood
Cloves
Equal parts, one teas spoon per cup 5X/wk for 1 month.

d) Bring in the good bugs

Use Bifa 15 from Eden foods
Use the most powerful probiotics your local Health Food Store has

Be careful - it will make you gas allot at first. I started with Bifa-15 because I liked it.

e) Boost your Immune System

Ed Skilling's Photon Genius

f) The Icing on the Cake

Hyperbaric Chamber - 2X/Wk one hour per session minimum.

Many folks sleep all night in their chambers.

We urge you to work with your local Health Care Provider - let us hope they are open to new ideas.

A special note to our GI's: There is hope. Even if you cannot afford the Hyperbaric Chamber or Ed Skilling's Machine using the other products seems to speed up the healing process tremendously.

In 1944 the U.S. Army did a test with wounded soldiers and found that those who were given proper nutrition (Hydroponics Veggies) healed twice as fast as those who ate Sea Rations.

We also buy as much Organic food as we can.

g) Clean out the Heart Plaque

Use Immusist

or

EDTA once per week

or

Eat Grass Fed Beef/Lamb only.

We do all 3 and when my heart that was injured in the service skips no plaque breaks off because I have NO plaque buildup.

That is a big Thanks to those products listed above.

Remember - star slowly: If it can help it can't hurt.

I hold no financial interest in any corporation, the FBI made sure of that when we put Russian Troops in Iran and seized 300 Nukes built by the USA for the Shaw of Iran and stopped the US/Iranian war in 2007.

When I recommend companies I do so because I believe in them and their products.

These US Soldiers coming back form the Gulf injured are my soldiers and they deserve the best I can provide for them.

Chapter Twenty-One

High Blood Pressure

There is a very simple solution to HIGH BLOOD PRESSURE and that is a stalk of celery each day. You will also find that Turmeric will even out your blood flow. Or you can virtually kill the fats from cooking oils by using cooking pots from Kitchen Kraft. (Both editors are using Kitchen Kraft cooking pots for this purpose.)

Chapter Twenty-two

Hyperbaric Chamber

The theory is that this Hyperbaric Chamber combined with an Oxygen Generator forces oxygen into the cells, kicking out diseases. There is a video actually showing Lyme Disease spiraling out of a Red Blood Cell.

The Chamber takes you down to 11 feet under water - that's all - but wow - what a rush - like a great cup of coffee for the rest of your life naturally.

So what else is it good for:

1) MS - There is a guy working near here full time who used to be in a wheel chair. Forty treatments later he went back to work.

There is a gal in my home town that was in a wheel chair and was told by her doctors to get some diapers because it is downhill from here. She went to 2 treatments per week and after 6 weeks was walking without a wheel chair.

2) Traumatic Brain Injury (And Alzheimer): after 40 treatments the brain is almost completely healed. Why every military hospital does not have 15 or 20 of these is beyond me.

Imagine the performance of the Infantry (Special Forces, Rangers) if each unit had 2 portable chambers with Oxygen Generators?

3) Swelling. Many Ambulances in Japan have these chambers as part of their normal treatment. This process forces air into a wound; thus reducing swelling and secondary injury caused by swelling.

Many folks use the chamber before an operation to reduce swelling after the operation.

4) Cerebral Palsy: There have been improvements after just 3 treatments. The local folks are still testing but results look good. The problem is - most CP patients do not have enough money to do 40 treatments and Medicare will not cover this machine - even though others who treat CP patients say it cures them. Apparently $4,000 is too much to put a person back to work.

They need to rethink their policy - the State and Feds need to treat people and make them well rather than string them along with drugs until they die.

5) Exercise: There are over 200 NFL Players who own one - it helps reduce pain after a workout, swelling decreases. Their Work Outs can be more intense.

Sylvester Stallone used the Chamber every day while working out for Rocky, it reduced pain so he could workout more.

6) Radiation Damage: Many feel that this chamber is the only way to heal tissue damaged by radiation.

7) Diabetes, Malaria, - the Literature is full of personal stories of how this amazing product works.

Treatment runs about $100 for a one hour session. We used the Vitaeris 320 with the Oxygen Generator. Total cost for the unit is around $28,000.

Consider the alternative -

If you need a small portable unit you can purchase the Solace for about $12,000.

How much better would your Olympic Athletes do if you had the 4 or 5 full scale Vitaeris Chambers with an Oxygen Generators for your athletes?

Many people sleep in these chambers. Tests show that after 40 treatments (2X/Wk) Adult Stem Cell Count is up 800%. Imagine how fast your athletes would heal if you used this chamber.

Many believe the increase in Stem Cells stops the aging process - time will tell. Either way - 12 hours later I still feel great.

You may purchase these at H3 Therapy at: 253-432-0022 FREE 253-432-0022 Or Bill at: 253-857-3220 FREE 253-857-3220 or 253-509-8552 FREE 253-509-8552.

CHAPTER TWENTY-THREE

MULTIPLE SCLEROSIS

Here are the "Cures," way to reverse MS:::::

a) Ed Skilling's Photo Genie. The cost is about $3,600 but it stops MS in its tracks - Period. See Skilling Institute.

b) Immusist. Start slowly - you have a lot of Toxins in your body. It will take several months to detox your body. So far tests show it is 100% effective. You will need about 1 bottle every 3 months. Cost: $33/mo. Go to Immusist.com.

c) The old tried and true. Use the Ion Cleanse on EBay - it runs $120 and you will sue one coil per month. Use this in conjunction with Immusist and WOW - you detox fast. It runs about 50 cents to detox for 30 minutes.

Also: Do not forget to have on hand Citricare from Vim and Vigor. I use 100 drops when I get sick and the next day I am always fine.

Also: See CURE FOR CANCER, UPDATE 3 (Chapter 7, page 50).

You have the right to be MS free.

When you are MS free share this with your doctor.

Before you begin any treatment ask GOD for HIS guidance. This is only a Guide Book and intended for your use.

When your MS begins to subside - do not thank me, thank the BIG GUY upstairs. I am only a messenger.

Cure for autism, Immusist, the Ion Cleanse, and Kelp.

1) First you must decide to live. Whatever your ailment you must decide that the modern medical community got you here - sick - so lets us look outside the "American Medical Box."

2) Begin with vitamins. We recommend you use Centrum Silver. Kelp is much better and if you can afford this then use it.

I personally found in me that Osteoporosis went away in 3 months, bone mass went from 65% - 105% in 3 months by using 1 Centrum every other day. VA records as shown on Ch 23 and 77 in Seattle.

3) Clean out your Liver and Kidneys with a tea of Burdock Root and Rose Hips. One teaspoon of each per week should do you.

4) To cure for cancer plus add iodine.

Chapter Twenty-four

Willard's Catalyst Altered Water

By Sir Dr. Will P. Wilson

http://disc.yourwebapps.com/discussion.cgi?disc=149495;article=142232

The later discoveries about regenerative discoveries evidently revealed that this combined solution will evidently cure all or most diseases as that the Dr. Willard's Catalyst Altered Water when used as a solution catalyst will increase not only the cellular oxidation factor by several hundred percent but also accelerate the absorption of co mixed additives like MSM (up to a thousand times and regenerate the human body to being longevity sustainable and approximate regenerative reversing the aging process to twenty years younger or more. This solution could be a means of leading to the discovery of human immortality as said by one researcher.

I have used Dr. Willard Catalyst Altered Water and other Catalysts to Regenerate Severed and Re-Attached Fingers within Four Days with a one hundred percent regeneration of this person's fingers.

In the middle 1990s I had been contacted in an event whereby a person who had accidentally cut three of their fingers off while they had been working at the Marriott Foods Plant that is located near Sea-Tac Airport in Seattle on a Saturday.

This person had contacted me crying and while still in a state of trauma after the surgery team affiliated with the Marriott Foods Processing facility had successfully micro surgically re-attached this person's fingers.

This was on a Saturday and I had been contacted in the early evening on this Saturday with this party asking me knowing that I know (things) what the average person could not even be capable of understanding.

They then asked me about what can I suggest to them to do under the circumstances so I replied that I will see them in the morning and that please do not tell anyone what I suggest for them to considering doing to soak their fingers in a solution that I will be putting together for them.

So I proceeded to do this: I secured a gallon glass jug, a Carlo Rossi wine bottle, that was sterile and I then filled it up with distilled water, and then I proceeded to do this: (All items Referred to here can be purchased on line).

Dr. Willard's Catalyst Altered Water

https://www.google.com/search?q=Dr.+Willards+Catalyst+Altered+Water&ie=utf-8&oe=utf-8&aq=t&rls=org.mozilla:en-US:official&client=firefox-a

The Complete Regeneration of Severed Fingers *within* Five Days Using Dr. Willard's Catalyst Altered Water combined with other Important Catalysts.

Board: http://disc.yourwebapps.com/Indices/149495.html

William Mount WILLARD WATER UPDATE 1 Mon Sep 3, 2012
http://disc.yourwebapps.com/discussion.cgi?disc=149495;article=142208;title=APFN

Dr. Willard's Catalyst Altered Water
https://www.google.com/search?q=Dr.+Willard%27s+Catalyst+Altered+Water&ie=utf-8&oe=utf-8&aq=t&rls=org.mozilla:en-US:official&client=firefox-a

Before you begin any treatment ask GOD for HIS guidance. This is only a Guide Book and intended for your use. What you do or don't do is up to you.

Chapter Twenty-five

List of Items Suggested

In previous pages

Burdock Root
Cinnamon
Rose Hips
Dandelion Root
Marshmallow
Artemisia Annua - Bitter Wormwood
Cloves
Bifa 15 from Eden foods

Use the most powerful Probiotics your local Health Food Store has.

1) Ed Skilling's Photon Genius
2) Turmeric - it stops the Growth of the Tumors Right Now!
3) Water Purification Tablets - Iodine.
4) Citricare - to knock back his Yeast Infection.

5 Centrum Silver Vitamins.
6) Immusist - to clean out his lungs.
7) EDTA - to clean out the blocked veins and arteries he now has. Yes - Eric does this too, just not as fast.

Chapter Twenty-six

Company Benefits:
Using Roth 401(k) and
Medical Savings Accounts (MSA)
to develop longevity of
Low Income Wage Employees

Written by: Sir Keith Ljunghammar

So your new job offers you medical coverage of various types; basic medical, dental, vision or comprehensive. Other medical benefits may cover extensive cancer coverage or a non-medical daily money coverage benefit when your income stops due to medical or disability ("Aflac"). Life insurance or daycare coverage may also be other benefits.

Beyond medical your company may also offer a 401(k) pension plan. This type of program is more generically referred to as a defined contribution program. You contribute with your own money. The money for your contribution is taken out prior to your receiving your paycheck. Another type of program is a defined benefit program.

Your years of service establish your benefits amount at retirement. Most companies use the defined contribution plans because the risk of investment responsibility and the return is under the employee's determination and not under the employer as is the case with the defined benefit program which is more common today.

All these benefits might seem to be "rosy" but watch out for the thorns.

What the company may not be telling you is your 401(k) benefit may not help your tax situation as commonly now thought as doing but your taxes may actually be higher later at retirement. But don't blame your employer; they are just trying to comply with their own pension plan rules so they can reduce their taxes. Your company employer HR (Human Resources) department is looking after the interests of top management and not your interests. Yes, HR does have a conflict of interest point of view here.

The real question you as an employee should be asking is; "What mixture of benefits and tax ramifications will maximize my tax return. Or put another way: What mixture of benefits and tax ramifications will minimize my tax liability. Those with little income and a huge Earned Income Tax Credit may need to concentrate on maximizing their returns while others with a small EITC amount may need to concentrate more on reducing their tax liability for their best overall return.

Benefits which may affect your income tax are: Reductions in Box 1 amounts on your w-2 (medical benefits and pension plan benefits generally), child care benefits paid by the employer may reduce your taxes, a child tax credit but only up to the amount of the tax liability. Likewise, Form 8880, may reduce your tax liability by ten, twenty or fifty percent of the amount contributed to your 401(k) but only up to $2,000 or a maximum of $1,000 tax credit or $2,000 if married filing jointly. Restrictions not mentioned and other conditions must be looked at as well. If you have children the Child Tax Credit may take off $1,000 per child. This would reduce most low income workers wages to zero by itself. The remainder if not used to reduce your taxes may add to your refund as well. Again here restrictions may apply. If your income is low your return will not reflect the refundable portion if < $15,000.

The dynamics of taxes and consideration of the use of company benefits keeps mounting.

Even though an Education Credit or better known as the Lifetime Learning Credit, American Education Credit or the Tuition and Fees Adjustment create additional dynamics to an income tax return and may help in reducing or eliminating an income tax liability. This will not be covered since it usually is not a company benefit and if it is the employer contribution amount to the employee may not affect the employee's income tax return.

Other avenues of tax reduction or tax deferment may be better handled by the employee and not by the employer benefit program however.

When it comes to contributing to a 401(k) plan or not the question answered may be to not contribute. But the real answer may be to contribute to your own retirement program in the form of an IRA or a Roth IRA. If your employer matches any funds you may be better off by putting your money into the employer's 401(k) plan rather than a traditional IRA. The employee decision to contribute may be determined by the employer's contribution amount.

The contribution to a Roth IRA comes into play when you can contribute and your tax liability is low or zero. You may not be able to lower your taxable income further with a Roth IRA but you will have control to take advantage of the Savers Credit after the end of the year when you have more control to figure the exact amount of contribution which you actually need to make.

Look at Form 8880 on *www.irs.gov.* In the upper right hand search engine section you will need to type in "Form 8880". (You can access all forms also by clicking on forms and publications in the left hand box at present in the middle of the page. All tax brackets are 50% of the contributed amount up to $200 or a $1,000 tax credit up to an adjusted Gross Income of $17,250. Single, MFS and Qualifying Widow(er) reduce down to 20% over $17,250 up to and including $18,750 and reduce down to 10% above this level to $28,750 when it goes to 0% above this.

Likewise HH is 50% to $25,875 then slides down to 20% until $28,125 and then 10% over $28,125 to $28,750. MFJ is 50% if not over $28,750. Above this level low income workers wages may not exist anyways. Double check your individual contribution amounts anyways to find out. See Form 8880 for further instructions.

Remember, the Savers Credit will only reduce your tax liability and the rest goes away or vanishes. Here is where you have the control with your contribution to your Roth IRA or traditional IRA after the fact with contribution by you where you do not with a 401(k) plan set up by your company as a benefit for you.

Congress made a big mistake here with 401(k) plans. They do allow companies to set-up Roth 401(k) plans but restrict the employee to making a set % to a 401(k) or Roth 401(k) plan at the point of hire. This potentially forces employees possibly to quit with their employment once per year to be able to control their defined contribution taxability contribution amounts for tax planning purposes. So they just offer one 401(k) program or a Roth 401(k) program. Usually the pension plan is a 401(k) plan because this defined contribution is more traditional, will reduce taxes, does not have upper income level contribution limitations and large companies like the plan administration although it is still cumbersome.

If an employer does offer a Roth 401(k) and your income is or is expected to be low and stay relatively low during your tenure or you will not be employed there long then their Roth 401(k) may be the defined contribution plan you are really seeking. Weigh your options but be truthful to your long and short-term financial situation.

Maybe some examples might help to better solidify the process you need to look for to help assure a sound tax return at next year's tax time.

First, some assumptions will have to be made. Your exact situation will invariably be different. It may be lower or it may be higher or it may be much higher.

Let's first assume you are single. For argument sake here we will also assume married filing separately status since most of the calculations for single and married filing separately are the same. The calculations for married filing separately as related to most tax credits and also to the EITC are disqualified for usage so separate calculations using married filing separately status will not be shown or calculated. Another little quark in the code is married filing separately status is disqualified for a Roth IRA due to not knowing what the spouses income would be. In essence this leaves the married filing separately taxpayer to accepting the pension plan of the employer. Ouch!

Married filing jointly, head of household, qualifying widow(er) do have some similarities but different tables and calculations are used on most credits so these filing statuses will be calculated separately later after looking at the single filing status.

The standard deduction for Single is $5,950.
The standard deduction for Married Filing Jointly (MFJ) and Qualifying Widow(er) (QW) is $11,900.
The standard deduction for Head of Household (HH) is $7,000.

Will be assuming an employee and the employees spouse are not dependents of anyone else as well. The income of a full-time employee and the option of an employer to disqualify pension benefits to anyone less than twenty-one will be assumed. Also assuming a worker is not a dependent of someone else. Since working full-time conflicts with education and being a full-time student at 21 to 23 years of age would limit a working taxpayer to a low income to qualify as a dependent above 23. This low income would have so many variables and another paper would have to be written by itself to cover all of the conditions.

The taxpayer employee is not a dependent.

Although a single person can have dependents but not be qualified under another filing status that is not a frequent occurrence and thus no dependents will be argued with the single filing status. A divorce and claiming a child every other year as a dependent can create this situation for instance. Also, an alien wife living abroad can create this situation with a statement of declaration included with the tax return.

Dependents or Personal Exemption amount will be calculated at $3,800. A taxpayer employee will have one personal exemption amount of $3,800. A spouse will have one personal exemption amount of $3,800. No age or blind test will be used to add value to a standard deduction amount.

Will be assuming the employee is working 40 hours per week for 52 week at a pay rate of $9.95 = $20,696.

Will be assuming the taxpayer receives a Child Tax Credit of $1000 when dependents are allowed. In the year the child reaches 17 the Child Tax Credit is not allowed.

Assuming medical will cost $20 x 52 = $1,040 or $25/week x 52 = $1,300 or $50/week x 52 = $2,600.

Assuming the taxpayer contributes 3% to a 401(k) plan and 20,096 x 0.03 =$620.88.

With no benefits and Single @ $9.95/hr.
$20,696 - $5950 (standard deduction) - $3800

(personal exemption) = $10,946 (taxable income)
Tax = $1,204.

With $20 medical benefit and single @ $9.95/hr.
$20,696 - $1,040 = $19,656
$19,656 - $5,950 - $3800
= $9,906 (taxable income)
Tax = $1,054.
A savings of $150 or 7.5 weeks savings from taxes is achieved.
$2.88 weekly tax savings.

With $25 medical benefit and single @ $9.95/hr.
$20,696 - $1,300 = $19,306
$19,306 - $5,950 - $3,800
= $9,616 (taxable income)
Tax = $1,009.

A savings of $195 and an additional savings of $45 for a total of 7.8 weeks savings of $25 - $20 = $5 medical cost difference. Weekly tax savings come to $3.75.

With $50 medical benefit and single @ $9.95/hr.
$20,696 - $2,600 = $18,086
$18,096 - $5,950 - $3,800
= $8,319 (taxable income)
Tax = $833.
Total tax savings of $221 for a total savings of $371 for a total of 9.4 weeks savings of $50 - $20 = $30 medical cost difference. This comes to $7.13 weekly tax savings.

With a 3% pension 401(k) defined contribution and no medical benefits and single @ $9.95/hr.
$20,696 - $620.88 = $20,075.12 - $3,800
= $10,325.12 (taxable income)
Tentative Tax = $1,114 - $62 (Savers Credit)
Total Tax = $1,052
Total savings compared with no benefit here is $152.

However, with an additional traditional IRA contribution of $1,946 - $620.88 = $1,325.12 an additional savings can be accomplished here. The reason is the Savers Credit jumps from 10% to 20% of the amount contributed.
$20,696 - $620.88 - $1325.12 = $18,750
$18,750 - $5,950 $3,800
= $9,000 (taxable income)
Tentative tax = $919 - $391 (Savers Credit)
Total Tax = $528.

Bringing your tax down from $1,204 to $528 = $676 tax difference. Contributing $629.88 + $1335.12 = $1,956 Retirement contributions = 1,956/20,696 = 10.58% retirement contribution.

With a not set in stone financial planning goal of ten to twenty percent retirement contribution amount this scenario is the first to accomplish that objective. Other criteria like your social security payment amount and the value of your house as an asset for retirement planning purposes or whether one will be living in their house for retirement must also be considered individually for ones own retirement life style.

An additional savings can be received by contributing an additional $1500 to your retirement plan(s).

$20,696 - $620.88 - $1,325.12 - $1,500 = $17,250
$17,250 - $5,950 - $3,800
= $7500
Tentative Tax = $753 - $1,000 (Savers Credit limited to tax liability)
Total Tax = 0

Total retirement contribution = $3,446 or 16.65%.
Since the maximum contribution possible is 15% to a 401(K) part of all of the contribution would have to be to a traditional IRA.

What would the results be if instead of a 401(k) the contributions were made to a Roth 401(k) or other Roth IRA.

The tax with no benefits is $1204. The income being $20,696 would result in no income reductions.

$620.88	$1,956	3,456 Contribution to retirement
1,204	1,204	1,204 Tax
-62	-196	-345 Savers Credit
Then		
$1,142	$1,008	$859 Roth IRA
Vs.	Vs.	Vs.
$1,052	$528	$0 Traditional IRA

The conclusion for single individuals without calculating out the combination of medical and pension 401(k) contributions is tax wise beneficial. The additional coverage for vision and dental can be justified by tax savings as contributions for medical coverage are not counted as taxable income.

Whether to have greater medical coverage is invariably up to the individual. A preventative program as described in Duke Bishop Captain Sir Dr. William B. Mount (U.S. Army, Retired) book "Cures Medical Experts will NOT admit to" may be a better and less costly path to take.

With the 10% tax rate for single's ending at $8,700 and the 15% tax bracket with an income over $8,700 but not over $35,350 it may be difficult to justify contributing to a 401(k) or traditional IRA just to get the tax liability down to zero. Funds would be tight. A Roth 401(k) plan to minimize end of life taxes and pay now rather than later may be justified. But contributing for single individuals to a 401(k) plan contribution might help their long term financial planning goals.

Another category would be married filing jointly. Daycare may come into play but only if both spouses are working or the other one is going to school or disabled and one is working. A Child Tax Credit of $1,000 will dramatically reduce a couple's income tax. In the single example medical and pension contributions combined did not equal a $1,000 tax reduction. Also, in most cases, the tax liability for single was barely over $1,000 at $1,204. With more dependents individual medical costs of $50 or more per week should be considered. A look for lower cost medical or an alternative MSA (Medical Savings Account) should be considered by the employee as well as by the employer. With lower costs in a group due to following Dr. Mount's protocols when symptoms do not exist (as a preventative measure) the employer will be able to build up a medical "pension" plan account and the employer will be able to enjoy longer term employee retention and lower medical coverage costs of the companies employee's. On the flip side of thesef employees should pursue an MSA/HSA (Health Savings Account) employer covered medical benefit when adhering to a pre-medical coverage protocol.

Since a Child Tax Credit may substantially reduce or eliminate any tax liability then a 401(k) plan to reduce a zero tax liability would be unfruitful and actually have a negative effect in the elder years. A Roth 401(k) plan or Roth IRA complimentary plan should be used instead. Employees may be free to move to other companies seeking employment if the employer does not provide a Roth 401(k) plan to MFJ employees during their time of low income producing employment years.

This is a strategy employees could be using. Also employers could be using the above strategy both for getting younger workers who might be more transient and adjusting the pension or medical benefits to attract and retain younger workers. Older workers may also be more attracted by medical coverage (MSA) and Roth 401(k) pensions due to their certainty of years and lower time value of money build-up as compared with tax differences.

Let's take a look at comparable married filing jointly examples. Married Filing Jointly will be assumed with one staying at home. Thus no day care will be calculated. In a two income earning family we cannot project how much the other spouse makes. If one spouse were going to school additional considerations to the American Education Credit, Lifetime Learning Credit or the Tuition and Fees

Adjustment could reduce the tax liability to zero without considering employment benefits. Since this paper is to compare employment benefits and determine any possible strengths or weaknesses which the employee or the employer can use or adjust so total overall changes on an employee employment or employer employment dynamic can be adjusted if needed.

Will be assuming one spouse makes $9.95/hr. No children for this scenario. No benefits received.

$20,696 - $11,900 (standard deduction) - $7600 (two personal exemptions) = $1,196 taxable income.
Total Tax = $119.

Here you can see that without calculating further medical benefits or a 401(k) plan would be of little benefit. With the $20 medical weekly cost amounting to $1040 and in the above example the total income being $1,196 or if $1,196 - $1,040 - $156 taxable income a ten percent tax to reduce could be simply be accomplished by having a $25/week medical cost benefit. Most non-working spouses should be able to suggest to the working spouse to use a family plan which would be ($50/month x 52 weeks = $2,600) a substantial medical benefit reduction. This reduces by itself the taxable income to zero.

To consider investing in a 401(k) plan for this employee would be ludicrous since the income could (due to a higher income at retirement) be taxed at retirement and no tax benefit is available currently. A Roth 401(k) pension plan would be beneficial but very little if any of a Savers Credit could be enjoyed either. A zero tax liability would be enjoyed here as well.

It might be if one spouse is seeking higher education while the other one works. No American Education Credit or Lifetime Learning Credit could be enjoyed or used either to any great extent.

The Tuition and Fees Adjustment would be of no benefit here either but might be the better choice when calculating out any possible Earned Income Tax Credit. But if the only option is earned income as compared to adjusted gross income and considering whichever is higher would be used to calculate the Earned Income Tax Credit in most cases except the lower income bracket then the Tuition and Fees Adjustment also would have no effect in getting a higher EITC but it would bring a lower taxable income which may be the only necessity especially with no children/dependents. With no children limitation the Tuition and Fees Adjustment could not reduce the Adjusted Gross Income enough to trigger an EITC. With one or two or three children the maximum EITC will be achieved as well and further reductions by reducing income from a 401(k) or traditional IRA would make no difference at all. The range to maximize EITC for one child is from $9,300 to $22,300 with an amount of EITC of $3,169. For two children an income of $13,020 to $22,300 will give $5,236 and for three children in the same income range as two children will give $3,891.

Contributing to a 401(k) or traditional IRA at this income level would not be beneficial except for the matching funds from an employer but upon distribution amounts plus the employer's contribution amount would be all taxed. A Roth 401(k) would be beneficial to an employee at this time. With a minimum matching by an employer of .75% for your 3.00% this is a twenty percent matching by the employer. You might be in the 15% or 25% tax bracket at retirement so without calculating the time value of money appreciation and the tax consequences of same I would forgo a 401(k) contribution and instead contribute to my own personal Roth IRA instead.

If I double my retirement plan then my overall taxes are on the whole with a 401(k) and still zero at retirement with a Roth IRA or Roth 401(k). I do not see the sense in locking in a tax liability when currently there is no tax liability. This would be true even if the employer offered a 100% matching funds contribution amount.

For Head of Household filing status I came up with a tax liability of $438 and no benefits, $338 with a $20/week medical plan, $63 with a 3% pension contribution and $0 with a medical ($20/week) and 3% pension contribution. Two personal exemption amounts were used because although not required to have a dependent in all circumstances most qualifying for head of household status do have at least one qualifying child or dependent. For instance, a divorce plan my specify every other year for the taxpayer claiming a dependent would be able to file under Head of Household status and care for a child to be able to also claim the child as a dependent. Daycare for a child when not claimed may reduce the tax liability here. Form 2441, if filed in advance, can rescind the divorce decree affect as well.

Other tax benefits like EITC still remain with the Head of Household taxpayer. The employee Head of Household taxpayer may want to maximize their EITC amounts but again to increase a 401(k) contribution just to decrease ones income and thus increase your EITC refund amount especially if your tax liability is zero currently does not make for sound tax planning.

The current maximum EITC for the Head of Household fling status is achieved in the $9,300 to $17,100 income range for an amount of $3,169 for one child. For two qualifying children the maximizing range is $13,050 to $17,100 with an EITC amount of $5,236. And a third child with the same income range as two the EITC amount is raised to $5,891.

In conclusion, the objective of the Human Resources Department (HR) is to work for the employer's interests. In order to attract highly skilled employees most employees by hiring necessity have medical and pension plans as benefits. Highly skilled individuals would continue to look for other employment or only use an employer as a short-term career if the basic two amounts are not offered in their company benefits package.

Also, most highly paid employees ($75,000) or higher in income may have their 401(k) contributions reduced after April 15th of the next year and have to adjust their tax return. Highly paid and highly compensated employees usually file extensions and build in large refunds so they can avoid any interest and penalty charges due to part of the 401(k) pension contributions being non-deductible. This can be more accentuated when a closely related group owns or controls more than 80% of the capital stock.

Except for the low wage single employee it is questionable if a 401(k) plan is advisable at all. A Roth IRA may be the best for contributions. This would be outside a company plan and thus would not receive any matching benefits. Only when matching benefits to a company sponsored 401(k) plan outweigh tax consequences. This would also be dependent upon how close one is to retirement and the years of employment required to have matching funds vested. Only when matching benefits to a company sponsored 401(k) plan outweigh tax consequences would this be beneficial. This would also be dependent upon how close one is to retirement and the additional years of employment required to have matching funds vested. Some companies vesting defined benefit programs range from instantaneous (profit sharing) to six years. All funds, whether vested or not are forfeitable if the employee takes anything from the employer. I guess Johnny Cash never did enjoy a pension plan from General Motors then either.

Employers should also look at alternatives to pensions as well. A healthy workforce may instead be less costly to an employer and a de-facto pension health care plan in the form of a MSA could be used after retirement through non-used employee medical accounts.

Restrictions, benefits and qualifications are uniform across all employee income classes (excluding as a union benefit) and thus special after-year ended calculations do not need to be made.

A healthier workforce produces more and thus costs less to the employer as well.

An employer who prominently hires low income wage earners may want to offer Roth 401(k) plans as an alternative to their 401(k) pension programs.

An employer who is seeking healthy employees may want to look at a MSA program for its employees. A healthy workforce lowers costs. A MSA also stimulates the employee to save or lower medical costs voluntarily due to the savings reverting back to the employee.

A healthy workforce though will lower the catastrophic medical expenses and thus could lower the employers overall medical expenses dramatically.

The conclusion is really to have tools available for what is the best for the overall employee.

The employer has various objectives and needs to keep in mind the expected usual longevity of employees, company hiring policies, legal constraints, age of closely held corporation members, marketing mix objectives, public relations, product packaging, price mix, vertical and horizontal integration of key products, cash flow, inventory movement, company hierarchy or companies with a greater than twenty percent ownership by member(s) of a closely held corporation and the other companies matching policy requirements, and other lesser requirements.

Good job hunting or great company longevity may be the standard operating procedure dependent upon how a company mixes its employee benefits package.

Chapter Twenty-seven

Cure your Finances by Establishing your Personal HSA or Health Savings Account

Chapter written by: Sir Keith Ljunghammar

HSA or Health Savings Accounts have benefits for both the employee and the employer. Flexibility, lowered cost, control of preventative measures, affective savings build-up for employee. The employer can benefit through their use of cafeteria plans which are addressed under Section 125 of the IRS Code. An HSA can discriminate towards highly paid employees with established procedures. Transfers risk from the employer to the employee especially with the use of cafeteria plans in my opinion. Employees have the control so risky lifestyles are reduced or eliminated by the employee and they can reduce their HSA account withdrawals or look for the best and least expensive medical coverage. A reduction of catastrophic expenses in a group would reduce employer catastrophic expenses for the group and thus allow the employer contribution amount to be lower or stable over time. A healthier happier employee base will ensue and retention of employees should be easier too.

What are some of the criteria, specifically, which the employer would need to look at for their best benefit?

The employer will need to address reporting requirements, such as:

1) Including contributions made to the employees HSA account and including on w-2, box 12, Code W and reported on other appropriate Forms sent to the National Government.
2) No government reporting required for establishing HSA accounts but only with a HSA trustee who would be with a qualified bank or insurance company.
3) Employment taxes would be reduced since amounts contributed are not considered as wages and thus would not be included on the employee's w-2, box 1, 3, or 5.
4) Anti-discriminatory rules are simple. See IRS Publication 969, page 10.

Comparable contributions If you decide to make contributions, you must make comparable contributions to all comparable participating employees' HSAs. Your contributions are comparable if they are either:

* The same amount, or

* The same percentage of the annual deductible limit under the HDHP covering the employees.

The comparability rules do not apply to contributions made through a cafeteria plan.

Comparable participating employees Comparable participating employees:

* Are covered by your HDHP (High Deductible Health Plan) and are eligible to establish an HSA,

* Have the same category of coverage (either self-only or family coverage), and

* Have the same category of employment (part-time, full-time, or former employees)."

""From IRS, Publication 969, page 10

Employers need to read and understand several items completely before deciding to establish a HSA benefit program. Under the search engine on the www.irs.gov home page include: Notice 200859, 2008-29I.R.B, 123 and see questions 23 through 27 or connect to the notices by using: www.irs.gov/irb/2008-29 IRB/ar11.html.

For employee comparability requirements for eligible employees see: IRS Regulation 54.4980G A-14(c).

Not adhering to regulations of comparability may result in an excise tax of 35% of the amount you contributed to the HSAs of non-comparable employees'.

Advantages for employees can be numerous.

Being associated with a group of fellow employees who have a direct benefit in lowering their medical costs by paying cash as an example to a physician for a discount and then sending the notice for payment to an account trustee can do lots to save money as well.

Yes, HSAs have "a higher annual deductible than a typical health plan..." IRS Pub 969, page 3. But it has "...maximum limit on the sum of the annual deductible and out-of-pocket medical expenses that you must pay for covered expenses. Out-of-pocket expenses include co-payments and other amounts, but do not include premium." An example of a Premium would be an out of area charge.

Under an HSA additional medical insurance without jeopardizing your eligibility can have coverage for; accidents, disability, dental care, vision care, and long-term care.

Additional insurance that provides for the following items is allowed:

* Liabilities incurred under workers' compensation law, tort liabilities, or liabilities related to ownership or use of property.
* A specific disease or illness.
* A fixed amount per day (or other period) of hospitalization.
Bullets* from IRS Pub. 969, page 4.

The regulation for contributions and maximum amount of contributions is currently $3100 and an additional amount of $1000 per year after turning 55 years of age is allowed.

If on Medicare your contribution amount is zero.

You can make contributions to your own HSA account through April 15th of the following year. If you make a contribution for the 2013 tax year then contributions made from and reported to the trustee for 2013 can be made from January 1, 2013 through April 15, 2014.

Your employer will report their contributions to your account on Form w-2, box 12, Code W. Employees cannot take an adjustment for the employer contributions on their Form 1040 tax return.

Partners in a partnership and S-Corporation contributions to a 2% or greater shareholder-employee HSA are included as adjustments on the Partners or S-Corp 2% or greater shareholder's Form 1040, line 25.

You will receive Form 5498-SA or 5498-HSA and along with your w-2, box 12, Code W amount you will include the employers contribution on your contributions on Form 8889.

If your combined yearly contributions exceed your HSA contribution limits then a 6% excise tax on excess contributions may need to be reported on Form 5329. If you pull this money out In a timely fashion along with the resulting increase from interest then this yearly tax may not apply.

Excess contribution of interest would be included on Form 1040, line 21 as "Other Income", and include the word 'HSA' as a marginal entry to the left of the dollar amount column.

Excess contributions to an HSA may be able to easily occur when 1) going form a family-plan to a self-only coverage, 2) spouse is eligible under employers plan and includes you under that coverage also, 3) loan encumbered plan, 4) becoming eligible for Medicare and getting the Medicare insurance, 5) taking out non-eligible insurance or some prescription drug plans, 6) becoming a dependent upon someone else income tax return, 7) establishing a non arms-length relationship with the HSA trust account, 8) working for two employers, 9) having non-qualified medical insurance coverage, 10) and other circumstances as mentioned in IRS Pub. 969.

Whatever you do respect the HSA account so you do not have to incur a 20% excise tax due to non-qualified withdrawals. The three exceptions for the 20% penalty are very specific. They are permitted due to death, disability or attaining the age of 65 of the account holder.

You should read IRS Form 8889 instruction booklet and Publication 969. Sections of Form 5329 pertaining to excise tax should be read as well. If you have excess employer contributions you may need to see the IRS Form 8889 instructions, page 6 and include "Filled pursuant to section 301.9100-2" at the top of your Form 1040 if you are required to retain your rights.

Now that you have the strength to control your personal medical condition through curing your ailments and diseases and can now control your costs or reduce your costs you need to inform your friends, relatives and co-workers of the same.

Inform your employer as well about their benefits and potential stabilization and/or reduction of costs of employee benefits through distributions of this book.

Have a Happy, Cured and Long Life.

Chapter Twenty-eight

Medical Round-up

Chapter written by: Sir Keith Ljunghammar

Now what really is the plan?

Your basics would be in following the directives for the chapter on Cure for Cancer, Update 3 (Chapter 7, page 50).

If you have looked at the chapter and some other aspects of the book you have realized there are some basics which should all be followed.

Here is a list of some of the basics. But do not exclude other suggestions of the book. Of course, always ask your pharmacist or physician about using the below. Some pharmaceuticals can interfere with the below. For instance, Turmeric will lower your blood pressure. If you are on a blood reduction medicine be very very careful. Iodine can be substituted with kelp tablets but you might be allergic to iodine if you have ever been on chemo-therapy. Substitute kelp tablets instead of using iodine. I use kelp tablets personally because they are easier to deal with anyways.

1) Vitamins. Take one Centrum Silver for men or for women. On the shelf you may find a less expensive vitamin. If you do substitute then substitute for a complete vitamin and mineral package. It is important to have a complete vitamin and mineral tablet. If there is only one thing you do then making sure a complete vitamin and mineral package is part of your goal should be your objective. Vitamins and minerals are essential for cell functioning. If essential vitamins and minerals are missing from your protocol then the other ingredients may be wasteful. Every other day may be all that is need. I take them every day if not just for my overall health.

2) Kelp tablets.

a) However, since most kelp is from Japan or Asia, use caution. Radiation from the Fukushima Nuclear Plant in Japan has seeped into the Pacific Ocean and continues to contamination the Pacific Rim. Check the label to make sure the kelp is not coming from the greater contaminated area.

b) Kelp is the substitute for iodine tablets. Caution, make sure you are not getting the 'for medical purposes' iodine. This can be extremely poisonous if continuously used. Surgeons use medical iodine to clean and sterilize a surface prior to surgery. You are not a surgeon but only need to get the tablet form and not the medical form of iodine. I get the iodine which can be found at an outdoor recreation store. I get the iodine which is used for purifying water when only stream or lake water is available. You should have these items in your house for emergency water purposes as well. Mix according to directions. Using the purified water with your green tea is one idea. But not too much iodine purified water should be used. At the most two cups every other day should suffice. Again, I use kelp because it is easier.

c) If you have taken or are on chemotherapy you will more than likely be allergic to iodine. Instead, substitute with kelp tablets which contains natural iodine. I personally prefer kelp tablets. Kelp and seaweed are virtually a staple in the Asian diet. Go ahead. It really does taste good in its natural form as well.

3) Green Tea. You may include half black tea if desired. I like just straight green tea or the green tea from "Dollar Store" with Honey and Ginseng added for my quick away-from-home drink. For only one dollar it certainly tastes great as well. Try not to add sugar and definitely do not include any artificial sweeteners. Sugar is a fuel for cancer and artificial sweeteners actually help in increasing your weight. Your brain is tricked and thinks you need more food.

4) Citricare. Fifteen to twenty-five drops per day. It is 'bitter' is an understatement. I usually take ten to fifteen drops once per week. I either put this into some type of a sweet drink or into my green tea. If you drink three cups of green tea in the morning perhaps try to put in five drops into each of the cups as you drink them. Funds lacking, Citricare may be the first thing to go. If you have a disease present and are not just using this protocol for daily maintenance then this is the first thing to be included along with your complete vitamins and minerals.

5) Turmeric. I take one tablet daily. The time I had skin cancer on my shoulder (diagnosed on May 4, 2012 and gone by the end of the month without the doctor using his scalpel) I increased the number of turmeric tablets from one to three per day. I also was taking fifteen drops of Citricare and increased my drops from fifteen to twenty-five after the first two weeks from diagnosis. I saw a dramatic increase in the reduction of the skin cancer after this increase. Also, no one can tell me this protocol does not work since it worked in me personally. I also saved $1400 in medical costs. Congratulate yourself ahead of time for your elimination of unnecessary expenses and scaring yourself for life.

6) Immusist. Immusist is absolutely powerful in clearing up the area around a cell. If you want to embark on health then Immusist must be in your arsenal of health intake tablets and/or drops. When AIDS/HIV is cured within thirty-five days on all African health cases (5000 of 5,000) it is noteworthy to include this ingredient. At about $100 per bottle for a sixty day drop supply of twenty-five drops per day I would take note. I never have taken Immusist but strongly recommend this for fast results.

7) EDTA. If you want to clean out your veins and arteries EDTA is one item which you should have. Remember Turmeric is a substitute for EDTA but slower in its results. With high blood pressure the sooner you get the problem licked the better. Continuing maintenance by continuing with EDTA or substituting Turmeric should be a personal health thought as well.

8) Decompression of hyperbaric Chamber Therapy. Here the objective is to increase the amount of oxygen getting to the cell

level or to the brain, depending upon your particular disease. By artificially taking one down to eleven feet below sea level for about fifteen to thirty minutes at about a $100 session visit your brain cells retains the oxygen at a higher rate. The oxygen fed into your system will help in triggering the healing process. PTSD, autism, Palsy and other nerve or brain originating diseases will be helped in the process. Athletes should also have some great benefits with this therapy as well.

PTSD and autism are two diseases which are showing extremely positive results as noted in prior chapters. Palsy does take up to seven years worth of treatments. Yes, expensive but worth it to say the least.

9) Ion Cleanse Machine. This machine will help in getting heavy metal garbage out of your system. Definitely a little bit of an investment. Some vendors have these machines at fairs or arts and craft shows. Try it and see how much garbage comes out of your system in just fifteen or thirty minutes. It is ugly. Continue to use monthly at a minimum.

10) Ed Skilling Photon Genius. If there is one medical process which should be used on virtually all medical diseases this is the one. But the cause or reason for the disease may still exist after usage. When one is extremely sick an instant cure to all diseases would be helpful. The Ed Skilling Machine does exactly that. About fifteen minutes and your disease is cured. If you can find a laboratory which has one of these take advantage of it. Think of the machine as the ultimate after-disease-vaccination cure without needle machine.

11) Inflammation. The objective of any cure is to eliminate the inflammation which is causing the disease. This creates a situation where minerals and vitamins cannot get to the cell level. Or perhaps you may need oxygen for the healing to take place.

Think again through to your solution.

Remember, taking Turmeric is a blood thinner and may affect other heart or blood-thinning medications. Check with your pharmacist or physician first.

12) Insurance. If you cannot become ill now why should you buy health insurance? In affect you are spending $3-5 per day for your medical insurance premium. The only additional medical insurance you may still need should be accident insurance. Accidents always happen and should be addressed through insurance. At $20 - $40 per month this is less than most employees matching medical insurance premiums. Or if you cannot do this look at the previous two chapters and then formulate your personal medical protocol and medical insurance solution.

What the above protocol does is:

1) Clears the intestines, veins and arteries.
2) Gets the ingredients to a cleaner intestine system where they can be absorbed into the body and cells by by-passing.
3) Cleans up the surrounding cell area so the cell can absorb the vitamins and minerals in a more efficient fashion. The normal inflamed cell absorbs about two to three or four per cent of the vitamins and minerals which are around the cell. Bring this number up to six or seven per cent and the cell will be able to

start to function as a cell is supposed to and thus the real healing process begins.

For additional information see Dr. Mount's instructions in the previous chapters. Also you may want to consult your physician and/ or pharmacists for further advice.

Keep in mind also that the 'Cure for Cancer' was actually discovered in 1947 by a United States Army study in Japan on the survivors of Nagasaki and Hiroshima. The citizens who did not take Miso soup and kelp passed away in two to five years. The one who did survived to a normal ripe old age. Evidently the radioactive heavy metals were "washed-out" of the body by these two ingredients. Fermented soy beans and kelp can be healthy after all. Or simply go to a Japanese Restaurant once per month and have Miso soup and some sushi.

Congratulations to your health.

61029704R00090

Made in the USA
Lexington, KY
26 February 2017